TurboCharged

TurboCharged

Accelerate Your Fat-Burning Metabolism,

Get Lean Fast

and

Leave Diet and Exercise Rules in the Dust

By
Dian Griesel and Tom Griesel

Foreword By

Fred Pescatore, MD, MPH, CCN
Author of *The Hamptons Diet*

Business School of Happiness Inc.
Washington Depot, CT

Copyright 2010

Business School of Happiness, Inc.
Attn: Permissions Dept.
P.O. Box 302
Washington Depot, CT 06794
860.619.0177
Published by Business School of Happiness Inc.
Cover Photos by Al Rodriguez
Editing by Judy Katz and Sebastian Thaler
Printed in the United States of America by createspace.

Business School of Happiness books and recordings are available through most bookstores as well as amazon.com. For further information, call 860.619.0177 or visit our websites at www.businessschoolofhappiness.com or www.turbocharged.us.com.

Substantial discounts on bulk quantities are available to corporations, professional associations and other organizations. For details and discount information, contact our special sales department.

PLEASE NOTE: The creators and publishers of this book are not and will not be responsible, in any way whatsoever, for the improper use made by anyone of the information contained in this book. All use of the aforementioned information must be made in accordance with what is permissible by law, and any damage liable to be caused as a result thereof will be the exclusive responsibility of the user. In addition, he or she must adhere strictly to the safety rules contained within the book, both in training and in actual implementation of the information presented herein. TurboCharged is a program for rapid body-fat loss. It makes no medical claims. It is the sole responsibility of every person planning to apply the techniques described in this book to consult a licensed physician in order to obtain complete medical information on his or her personal ability and limitations. The instructions and advice printed in this book are not in any way intended as a substitute for medical, mental or emotional counseling with a licensed physician or healthcare provider. Before beginning the TurboCharged program, we suggest that when you consult your physician you request a complete physical along with full blood-panel testing. These numbers will serve as an excellent baseline to measure your progress as you follow this program.

ISBN # 978-1-936705-00-9
Library of Congress #2010918143

This book belongs to: _____

DEDICATION

Dian: To Rory, Chamonix and Steel

Tom: To Janet and Joe

Dian and Tom: To Our Mom Jane

In Memory of Jack LaLanne

*"What does age mean?   Not being able to do the things you used to do.
If I can get you doing things you haven't done for years, isn't that exciting?"*

September 26, 1914 – January 23, 2011

TABLE OF CONTENTS

Acknowledgments

We'd like to thank our families, especially our spouses Janet and Rory, for all their loving care, patience and advice, especially during this process.

We'd like to thank all of the people who experimented with us, especially those who allowed their stories to be shared in these pages.

Thanks to Dr. Fred Pescatore for contributing the Foreword. Please go to his website (www.hamptonsdiet.com) and read his many excellent books that cover everything from weight loss to asthma to creating healthier children.

Thanks to all who participated in early readings of this book and offered their suggestions and immensely valuable advice.

Thanks to the countless CEOs, medical and scientific officers, researchers, medical doctors and others who have shared their scientific research and developments with us while participating in healthy debate.

Thanks to Judy Katz for being a true friend and brainstorming collaborator.

Thanks to Sebastian Thaler for his editing talents.

Thanks to J. Kevin Moran, Vice Admiral, USN retired, for managing IRG so efficiently and getting us in "ship shape" which allowed the time and support to complete this book.

Thanks to all of our friends who have let us talk endlessly as we have formulated our theories and debated their merits. You all helped make this a better program.

Finally, thanks to everyone we haven't listed here…you know who you are. We appreciate your love, encouragement, support and friendship.

Foreword

When I first read *TurboCharged*, two thoughts came to my mind. The first was that I myself am TurboCharged, and I felt really excited about that. My next thought was: "Wow! Look how easy it is to lose weight, and more important, maintain a healthy weight!" Indeed, Dian and Tom have written a book that is not only for those who need to shed pounds but also for those who want to keep it off, live a long life and reduce their biological age. Consequently, I believe the book can significantly improve the health of the general population.

Being a doctor who practices nutritional medicine, I have seen patients gain and lose perhaps millions of pounds throughout the course of my career. I firmly believe it is possible to lose weight by following any weight-loss program. As Dian and Tom point out, if you are overweight, you are consuming at least 3,500 calories per day—far more than is necessary for most people. Therefore, any diet program, no matter how you carve it out, will have you eating less than that.

So you lose weight and then the diet stops. Most people will then go back to eating the way they did before, because food means so much more to us than merely a means of fulfilling the energy requirements for our "vehicle." And before you know it, you have gained back the weight you lost and then some. *TurboCharged* does an excellent job at helping you to fight those feelings and live in cruise control mode.

Although I have written multiple diet books and coach hundreds of people on a weekly basis about their battle with food, the concepts of how to lose weight are simple— and *TurboCharged* couldn't make them any clearer. I found myself reading the book more and more quickly as the day progressed. It was turbocharging the way I read.

In all seriousness, we live in a society where we are quite literally eating ourselves to death. At least four of the top 10 leading causes of death can be linked to the lack of nutritious food in our diets. The less nutritious the food, the more we want of it. We are stuffing our faces with calories and our bodies are starving for critical nutrients. We are on a very dangerous path.

Dian and Tom describe very complex metabolic pathways and hormonal balancing as simply as possible. And I don't say that negatively. It is refreshing to have a diet book written by two highly motivated individuals who are simply saying: "Look, the science may be tough to grasp, so don't worry about it; here is what you need to do, here is why you should do it, and here are the results you should expect." For two people who do not hold medical degrees, their grasp of the science and most importantly their presentation to the reader is unsurpassed in diet books.

Everyone wants to "lose weight," but what we *really* want is to lose fat, or more precisely, shrink it—because once you have acquired a fat cell, it is there for life. The focus is always on the number on the scale, but *TurboCharged* puts the emphasis on your body-fat percentage—a true indicator for increasing your health and lowering your risk for certain food-related diseases, such as heart disease and stroke.

The authors' concept of the land of Leandom and the highway traveling there is a fantastic way to present what every one of us ultimately wants: to be lean and healthy. It is important to emphasize, as the authors do, how we originally ate during Paleolithic times. Our diets remained relatively constant until about 120 years ago; since then, they have changed dramatically, and we have gotten fatter because of it. Our genetic makeup just doesn't have the capability to change as quickly as the menu at your favorite fast-food restaurant. While 120 years may seem like a long time, it is but a nanosecond in evolutionary terms. *TurboCharged* takes us on this historical journey and makes it relevant for how we live our lives today.

Dian and Tom may have some controversy on their hands with their "no grain is a good grain" approach. It is a daring idea to write about, and I applaud them for doing so. I haven't eaten grains in years, since I believe they are the reason why we are so sick. I also think the proponents of grains, such as large agribusiness and big pharma, have an agenda. (Who do you think funds the studies that conclude that grains are healthy?) Keep the population sick and over-fed with too many calories but insufficient nutrition and it is a win-win for the largest companies in America and the world.

I digress a bit, but *TurboCharged* brings out that rebel in me. It emphasizes water, which is so crucial for health and fat loss. It tackles the exercise industry—why spend so much time doing it when you only need a few minutes several times per day? Move, people! Eat real food! Stop obsessing about carbohydrates/fats/proteins/salt, etc. Can it be any simpler? After reading *TurboCharged* you will know that it's not rocket science to lose fat and get healthy.

I think the problem with many diet books is that the emphasis is on teaching the reader why they are doing what they are doing. While *TurboCharged* does that, it is a book that really doesn't bog you down. It tells you what to do, when to do it, and if you follow the very simple guidelines, you too will be dropping fat, leaning out and attaining your goal of a lower body-fat percentage, decrease in inches and a younger metabolic age. *TurboCharged* is a system designed with our genetics in mind, based on sound science. With a combination like that, you can't fail.

Fred Pescatore, MD, MPH, CCN

Author of *The Hamptons Diet*

Authors' Preface:
A Note to Men, Women, Carnivores, Vegetarians and Cafeterians:

We appreciate high-performance cars. Aston Martins, Corvettes, Porsches, Ferraris, Maseratis and Lamborghinis are unique, exquisite and beautiful. People stop and stare. We are all in awe of these exotic machines. They capture our attention because their bodies are sleek, powerful and sexy. If you actually owned (or own) one of these beauties, we bet you would take really good care of it. You would keep it clean and in perfect running order using only the best parts, oil and gas that money can buy. But most of all, you would get it out on the road, show it off and drive it fast!

Why, you may ask, if this is a rapid fat-loss book, are we talking about cars?

You may or may not ever own an exotic car, but guess what? You already own something that is more wondrous and mechanically far superior to anything that will ever be designed: the human body.

Your "vehicle" may need a tune-up to get it into sleek, powerful, sexy and awe-inspiring condition. Here is where this book comes in.

You are now holding in your hands a significant chapter from the official owner's manual for the most important, high-performance mode of transportation on Earth.

Fasten your seat belt and hold on to your hat as YOU
prepare to lose excess body fat *FAST.*

Get ready to be TurboCharged.

Introduction:
The TurboCharged Promise

The TurboCharged steps as presented in this book will out-perform any other diet or exercise program you may have tried in the past. For many, this simple program will mean finally getting a sleek, healthy body for the first time after a lifetime of disappointment. Yes, these are bold statements— but not unsubstantiated. Anyone, regardless of age, can do this. We guarantee you will see results on the scale and in the mirror in inspiringly record time while your moods and spirits begin to soar. After all, losing body fat quickly, while improving your health, is a naturally great mood elevator. It will be very easy.

Three days is all it will take to start your body and spirit racing toward a lifetime of lean. ***Within 10 days or less***, you will be convinced. There are no gimmicks, supplements or special ingredients required. There is nothing to buy. This book shares everything you need to get going on your personal road to success.

TurboCharging leads your brain to source excess body fat for energy instead of muscle, cookies or that bag of chips. Your brain gets comfortable as you follow the steps as presented. It realizes there is plenty of stored fat just waiting to be consumed because your body will be receiving plenty of nutrients from all the foods you will be eating. In just a few days, this so-called "diet" is perceived as no diet at all. You are suddenly TurboCharged. Your brain no longer reacts as if it is facing the stress so common to typical dieting. The new way you will learn to flex your muscles elevates your metabolism and your brain is directed to a bountiful new energy source: YOUR BODY FAT!

TurboCharged works, and keeps on working for us, for those whose stories you will read about in these pages and for countless others who have been coached through these eight simple steps. This is not a typical diet book. We will not be providing meal plans or recipes. We will, however, give you all the information and know-how you will need to lose not weight—which is comprised of water, bones, fat and essential organs and tissues—but excess body fat, which is the only thing you want to lose. In the process, you will reset your metabolism on multiple levels: You will have increased the number of calories you need to fulfill your daily activities—meaning you can eat more; you will have decreased your metabolic age; and you will have essentially improved your overall health in the process. People of all ages have tried TurboCharged and astonishingly, 100% of them reported amazingly rapid loss of excess body fat that was far beyond their most ambitious expectations. You will read about their experiences in their own words. A success rate does not get any higher than 100%.

Especially unusual, although not unexpected, is that the over-50 age group reports unanimous success in dropping all their unwanted extra body fat through this program. These are men and women who had tried pretty much every diet program and meal plan available and always, if they lost anything, gained it right back plus more. Over time, they had all become resigned to not losing weight because of their age, hormones, lack of physical activity or the constant stress in their lives. Nonetheless, while TurboCharging, they rapidly began losing the 20 to 50 or more extra pounds they could not shake off with other programs. Their excess body fat was lost so quickly, they could hardly believe it possible. Many TurboChargers report body fat percentages only achieved by top athletes. More interesting, they claim to have faster metabolisms—stating they now eat more than ever, yet maintain their new physiques that somehow continue to improve with minimal effort. TurboCharged works for everyone!

We will begin in Step #1 by dispelling most if not all conventional diet and exercise advice that you may have read about in magazines, newspapers or books, seen on television or the Internet, or heard on the radio from countless medical doctors, dieticians, nutritionists and other health care professionals. You will quickly learn that Turbocharging breaks all the rules that you may "know" about weight loss.

In Step #2, you will learn how you can begin charting your progress by tracking how your body fat is decreasing—not loss of water and muscle like other programs. Equally thrilling, you will learn how to document that your metabolic age is decreasing! Imagine how you might feel if you could see—without any drugs, injections or surgery—that you have accessed your own personal Fountain of Youth. We, Dian and Tom, can assure you, this is more inspiring than you can presently imagine. For example, let us tell you that according to the calendar Dian is 50 and Tom is 57 years of age, yet our base metabolic ages as calculated now show us to be 17 and 18, respectively. Our body-fat levels are at 13.5% for Dian and 10% for Tom. We are each in the best shape of our lives—stronger and leaner than our high-school years. (Our individual journeys to becoming TurboCharged are offered at the end of this book.)

TurboCharging not only allows you once and for all to lose your excess body fat quickly, it also reduces your metabolic age and improves all of your essential biomarkers. Likewise, your skin tone will improve and your energy will soar. Strangers will compliment you on your appearance and you will receive plenty of extra attention from your family and friends. The rewards will be quite visible.

In Step #3, you will learn about the only true fat-burning elixir and it's free! Step #4 will teach you all about how to use something you already do every single day to your rapid fat-loss advantage.

While eating foods you know and love, you will be building muscle and strength via the release of your hormones and other growth factors that are triggered by the steps we will soon share. You will achieve this with no exercise at all in the traditional sense of the word, as you will soon learn in Steps #5 and #6.

Each of these pages unfold to offer logical and easy time-tested principles that work *with* your body's natural rhythms. In Step #7, for instance, you will learn why in the past your willpower was strong until the late afternoon or evening. More importantly, you'll learn how to work *with* this natural urge instead of fighting against it. You will also learn which foods best help you reach your personal objectives and stay in the Winner's Circle forever. Step #8 explains how you can "see" your goal, by learning simple techniques that deliver a more relaxed state of mind and pleasant moods that help propel you toward your goal. We will show you, once you have reached your ideal level of body fat and a perfectly toned body, how to easily keep it in Cruise Control for life. We also have an extensive question-and-answer section that should resolve any part of this program that might still need clarification for you.

With TurboCharged we have both "connected the dots" and introduced new unique concepts to create a best-of-the-best paradigm for rapid fat loss, while eliminating all the unnecessary fluff and jargon. We have purposely made this book high on simple directions and suggestions, while low on science. We have found most people we meet simply want to know "how" to do it, not necessarily "why" it works. If you'd like to learn more about the plethora of science supporting "why" *TurboCharged* works, please take the time to go to <u>www.turbocharged.us.com</u> to read the hundreds of references we have posted. You can also refer to the Supplemental Reading List at the end of this book.

Getting TurboCharged is for anyone who wants to be in better shape—including those who are already active and in good shape, yet still desire to improve their appearance and athletic performance. Accordingly, the athletes who have followed the TurboCharged steps reported to us that they achieved both subtle and quite obvious improvements that were previously unattainable. In fact, active people who have spent their lives exercising rather than dieting and who thought their weight and body-fat levels were just fine have relayed to us that they had no idea what dramatic improvements they could make to their health, well-being, appearance and performance until they committed to TurboCharged. Several have shared their stories in these pages.

Your Turn

Now it is your turn to join us on this wondrous TurboCharged adventure. To make sure we have your full attention so you can get the maximum benefit, we have a few simple requests. Please,

- Keep an open mind—at least until the end of the book. Suspend all of your pre-existing beliefs about diet and exercise, as you take in what this program can impart.

- Read the book from beginning to end before starting to work the program. By the end, it will all tie together and make perfect sense.

- Own the book. It is yours and yours alone. If your friends or family are interested in what you are reading or doing, please encourage them to invest in their own copy to read and keep as a valuable resource as well.

- Reread sections as you need to, in order to reinforce your understanding, intention and day-to-day commitment. And last but not least,

- Agree to focus not on losing weight but on losing excess body fat, with the expectation that you can become lean, possibly for the first time in your life.

While you contemplate this pledge to yourself, here is our pledge to you:

We, Dian and Tom, do hereby pledge that we do not have any hidden agenda other than spreading health via leaner bodies and happier beings. Yes, we'd love for you to recommend this book to others, but please be assured that we have no allegiances to any employers, government agencies, professional licensing boards, sponsors or other powers that could in any way compromise our clear message about decreasing your excess body fat and increasing your health! Instead, we have put together some definitive conclusions drawn from our years of accumulated research in addition to plenty of personal trial-and-error experimentation.

As with all things in life, to profit from any new idea, you need to be open-minded and ready for a change. If the time is right for you—and since you are reading this we would like to believe it is—if you in fact are, right this moment, at the point in your life where you genuinely seek freedom from excess fat, obesity and disease, then please take responsibility by educating yourself and seeking the truth. Don't buy into fad, fantasy or socially accepted dogma, as so many do. Take a look at the overweight and obesity statistics. Do they indicate that most people are on the right path, despite all the books, articles and diet programs? We think not!

We have taken our stand against the traditionally accepted concepts regarding both diet and exercise because they are clearly not working. There has to be a better and faster way. A direct route. There is. This is it.

Step #1
Forget What You've Been Told
About Dieting

If the numbers on your scale and a look in the mirror tell you you're overweight, you've probably tried at least 10 different diets with greater or lesser degrees of success. Yet here you are, reading another book.

There are hundreds of diets designed to attract the hopeful, but given the poor results, clearly something major is missing in this cornucopia of professional advice. We are a fat nation despite the fact that we have more gyms, more diet foods and more diet books than any other country in the world. Search Amazon.com for "weight loss" and you will see a whopping 16,881 diet books listed. So why are we bothering to write book #16,882?

Two reasons:

First, TurboCharged is a holistic program in which no one part stands alone. It is the combination of all its aspects that will provide you with a new way of attaining a lean, healthy body for life.

Second, TurboCharged is proven to be 100% percent successful for those who follow the eight simple steps. As we mentioned earlier, every single person who committed to TurboCharged for the initial 10 days to get started reported that the results were far beyond their wildest expectations. All of them kept going and continue to stick with the TurboCharged program today. It is that easy. They might waver occasionally, but they quickly get back in the driver's seat and stay the course.

Before we discuss the most common myths that play havoc with your intentions and have likely caused numerous crashes in the past—despite your best dieting intentions—please look at this list. Check off any that best reflect your motivation to get lean and healthy once and for all.

❐ You have been told by your doctor that being over-weight puts you at risk for high blood pressure, heart attack, high cholesterol, Type 2 diabetes, metabolic syndrome, cancer, sleep apnea, osteoarthritis, gallbladder disease, fatty liver disease, allergies, shortness of breath, joint pains, and more—any and all of which can shorten your lifespan and impact the quality of your life.

❐ You want to live to enjoy your children and grandchildren.

❐ You want to lose weight to fit into your outfit for a special event.

❐ You want to look good for your high school or college reunion.

❐ You are sick and tired of being fat, sick and tired.

❐ You are a fit, yet fat, person, and you don't understand why.

❐ You want to enhance your athletic performance.

❏ You want to be more attractive to potential partners.

❏ You want to improve your appearance to attain a better job or more clients.

❏ You want to enjoy your life much more than you are enjoying it now.

❏ You'd like to look in the mirror (naked or not!) and love what you see.

Whatever brought you to read *TurboCharged*, welcome. Sigmund Freud said there are no accidents, that everything happens for a reason, even if we don't always know what that reason is. What is important is that you are here. Let's begin working together by clearing up some common, yet quite serious, diet and fitness misconceptions. Any one of these could wreck your "vehicle" when it comes to fat loss and achieving your ideal body composition.

Some Common Myths Keeping You From Your TurboCharged Goal

☠ Weight loss equals fat loss. (Definitely not true, and a scary thought.)

☠ Eat a big breakfast to start the day right. (Wrong. Might even halt fat loss.)

☠ Five to eight smaller meals per day are best. (Maybe true, depending on the meal.)

☠ Exercise 30-90 minutes for maximum fat-burning benefits. (Sounds exhausting to us.)

☠ Balanced meals with protein, carbohydrates and fat are best. (Only if you like indigestion!)

☠ Grains are a necessary part of a balanced and healthy diet. (Not true.)

☠ It's best to sip water throughout the day. (Why?)

☠ Heavy weight lifting is a must for burning fat. (Not true, and might slow it down.)

☠ Fat-burning supplements are helpful. (False, and may even be dangerous.)

☠ High-protein, low-carbohydrate diets are best for weight loss. (No fruit? How horrible!)

☠ Eating fats will make you fat. (Not true. What kinds of fat are we talking about?)

☠ A high-carbohydrate diet is best for energy. (What counts as a "carbohydrate"?)

☠ A moderately low-calorie diet is best. (If you want to take forever to get lean.)

☠ A 1-2 pound weight loss per week is best. (Not true, and that might take a long time.)

☠ All calories are the same. (Really? Says who?)

☠ Glycemic Index diets work. (Not necessarily true. What about Glycemic Load?)

☠ Very low-calorie diets are bad. (Might be true…depending on what is eaten.)

☠ Sports drinks and fruit juices are good for you. (Not true if you want to get lean.)

☠ Protein or high-carb snack bars are nutritious meal substitutes. (Absolutely not true.)

Confusing, right? It's no wonder we are getting fatter despite our best intentions.

Why You Can't Win with Traditional Diets

There are three things most diets have in common: low calories, aerobic exercise and ample carbohydrates like beans, grains, rice, tortilla wraps, other bread sources, nutrition bars and sports drinks for energy. Breaking it down further, the "low-calorie diets" typically consist of 1,400-1,600 calories a day and sugar in its assorted forms as a constant ingredient; and participants are required to do 30-90 minutes of aerobic exercise and intensive weight lifting at least three times per week. Any diet with these combined recommendations will ultimately result in failure and disappointment. We will explain why.

If you are overweight, chances are you are used to eating at least 3,500 calories a day. Simple logic tells us that, if you decrease daily calorie consumption by 2,000 calories a day while also stressing your body with aerobic exercise as prescribed, you are creating a serious energy deficit. Your brain starts screaming and complains loudly: "You are starving me! I'm feeling very grumpy now! I want more sugar! Feed me!"

Any traditional program, like all of those on the preceding list, that reduces calories, adds heavy exercise yet is still sugar-centric, causes your body to quickly retreat into survival mode. It will reregulate your metabolism to continue functioning at the reduced caloric intake levels, and often accomplishes this by converting your lean muscle mass into fuel for energy. So while you may be "weighing" less, you are getting flabbier or just "shrinking" at the same time. Obviously NOT the way to win any race! Compounding this frustration is the fact that if a person's body rebounds and becomes overweight again by a certain number of pounds, that weight will become a new set point. It then becomes increasingly difficult to maintain a lower weight. Dieters know this. They call it the "yo-yo" syndrome. They experience it and cry: "After I stop dieting it seems like every mouthful I eat turns into more fat." Sadly, they are right. Traditional dieting that reduces calories, adds aerobics and has your body running on sugar for energy ultimately causes more and more fat to be hoarded by your body.

The next serious roadblock that cannot be ignored is simply the time it takes for success. The typical dieting scenario goes something like this: "I need to lose 20 pounds. So at a pound a week, if I start on New Year's Day, and I stick to my diet and find the time to exercise 30 to 90 minutes five days a week, by Memorial Day Weekend I'll fit into my bathing suit."

We say, "Red Light! Stop! Do Not Proceed!" That old routine represents a lot of hunger, deprivation, sore muscles and grumpiness for a mere 20-pound weight loss and five months of grueling work and bad moods. Pull in for a pit stop and let's talk about recharging your batteries with a whole new way of thinking.

The Key to Rapid Body-Fat Loss

The basic essence of TurboCharging is learning how to keep your muscles strong and vital in just minutes each day, while simultaneously retraining your metabolism to call for excess body fat as its primary fuel source.

To supply your body with its preferred fuel source, excess body fat, TurboChargers practice what we call enlightened fasting. Enlightened fasting has nothing to do with starvation or fasting by any traditional definitions. Starvation is bad for you and certainly not ever recommended. Fasting in the true sense of the word should only be done with strict medical supervision. Enlightened fasting, however, is great! Enlightened fasting, done the TurboCharged way, accesses excess fat reserves. It uses this excess fat for energy until those fat stores are depleted. During the entire time, you will still be eating plenty and nourishing your body with delicious and tasty foods.

Enlightened fasting is actually a whole new take on starvation. TurboChargers starve our bodies of those foods that trigger high insulin release. We have learned that any extra body fat has prepared us well for a little enlightened fasting, and, as a matter of fact, "fasting" (or in this case starving the body of damaging insulin spikes) is a very good thing.

History and science prove that limited periods of enlightened fasting the TurboCharged way:

- Have been practiced by humans and animals since the beginning of time.

- Restores hormonal balance and allows the body to clean out and eliminate accumulated waste and fat.

- Is the key to restoring cell vitality.

- Is the best defense against aging (along with not smoking!).

- Will return you to a TurboCharged body that gets to lean easily, stays there with minimal effort and works like an efficient machine with optimal functioning.

TurboCharged has proven countless times that eating plenty of natural and healthful foods that limit insulin production in the body, along with following the other steps outlined in these pages, will safely, easily and quickly deliver rapid loss of body fat. At the same time, you will be building muscle tone and shape almost effortlessly. Side benefits include improvements in blood pressure, diabetes if you have it, bone mass, allergies, sleep, skin, stamina, joint pains, mood and attitude.

You, like other TurboChargers, will find you have an exciting new level of motivation as you watch the scale drop three or more pounds of body fat every four to five days. It is thrilling to see how your clothing becomes looser while your new eating habits become automatically integrated into your routine. TurboCharged is simplicity itself, and rapid results are all the inspiration you will need to keep going all the way to the finish line.

Nutritionally complete, with more nutrition per calorie than virtually any other diet ever created, TurboCharged foods are not low-carbohydrate or low-fat. They are not high-calorie or low-calorie. This is not about high or low protein. As you will learn, it is the perfect way to eat for the rest of your life. The TurboCharged foods and the ways you will learn to eat them will simply help you feel full and satisfied while eliminating all the usual diet-related psychological stress. Once you are TurboCharged and have reached your goal, your metabolism will continue to burn energy efficiently to maintain your new sleek and lean body.

While delivering higher levels of body-fat loss, TurboCharging will also produce favorable physiological profiles. You will see improved glucose values with increased glycemic control for diabetics. Cardiovascular risk declines as blood pressure lowers, along with fasting glucose, total cholesterol, low-density lipoproteins (bad LDLs) and triglycerides. Regular follow-ups with TurboChargers have found these are lasting results with no return of body fat. We encourage you to discuss all of these points with your doctor, as this will be YOU!

You can see how certain misinformation may have prevented your success in the past. Let's move on to Step #2 and learn how TurboChargers measure performance and results. Knowledge is power. The power you need to live life sleek, lean and healthier lies just ahead.

An Amateur Cyclist and Exceptional Athlete Gets TurboCharged

Scott Savin, 51, is an elite amateur cyclist with the self-discipline and focus that allow him to push his mind and body to perform in ways that few non-professional cyclists can match. He rides under extreme conditions and extreme temperatures with as much as a 20-below-zero wind chill factor.

By day he's a consultant in the real estate business. As a cyclist he rides up to 15,000 miles and has climbed as much as 850,000 vertical feet in a year. He's been riding for over 32 years and jokes, "I have more than 600,000 miles on my legs." (Don't we wish our cars could do that!)

In July 2009, Scott carried 188 pounds on his six-foot frame, with body fat of 21%, too much weight and body fat for a cyclist of his caliber.

"Even with all of my extensive training and grueling competitive races, my weight never dipped below 181 pounds and my body fat held in the 21% range," says Scott.

Tom explained to Scott how TurboCharged worked, and gave him the program outline. "If you faithfully follow the program for just three weeks, you will unquestionably reach what you now think are impossible goals," Tom promised.

Scott admits that he was skeptical. "Another yada-yada diet," he thought. "However, in three weeks my total weight was down to 168 pounds with 12% body fat. My waist is now 32", a full five inches smaller than it was three weeks before. Unreal!"

Best of all, Scott has kept his excess fat off. "And what's even more exciting," he says, "I never lost any strength as I lost body fat, and my cycling times have actually improved by 15 percent."

In reviewing his TurboCharged accomplishments, Scott feels that although his body was a great calorie-burning machine, he apparently was not metabolizing his food properly. When he followed the TurboCharged steps and stopped eating all of the concentrated carbohydrates like pizza, pasta and bread, routinely recommended to high-octane athletes, he lost weight and body fat while increasing his performance at the same time.

Scott sums it all up: "I wish I knew how to TurboCharge 20 years ago. I've been on every diet and every fat-burning program that exists, and I know this one is the healthy cure for obesity we've all been waiting and praying for. With TurboCharged, the long wait is definitely over. I hope everyone learns about TurboCharging and gives it a try."

Step #2
Measure REAL Success

Back to the problem with those thousands and thousands of diet books: 99.99% include one nearly universal and MAJOR flaw.

In the many diet books you've read, do you recall any of the authors telling you to go out and buy a body-fat scale? Or did they just tell you to weigh yourself once a week to chart your progress and not any sooner than that so you don't get disappointed. Why do they say this?

Let's get to the first thing you most likely have never learned from a diet book. From now on, you are going to measure your success in one way and one way only: a decrease in the percentage of your body fat. We will show you how.

A common practice among dieters, nutritionists, nurses, dieticians and medical doctors is to track progress with common weight scales. Since lean muscle tissue is 15% denser than fat, higher weight loss, which might actually be loss of your lean muscles, is applauded. This is the antithesis of our measure of health and success.

The use of weight scales, coupled with not calculating body-fat percentages, is likely the root of all the conflicting studies, clashing theories and multiple "weight-loss" directives that have been keeping you from the finish-line prize of a sleek, lean physique. Even the new directive by the Obama

Administration requiring doctors to record our Body Mass Index (BMI) along with height and weight measurements is just plain useless. It only serves as more proof that so much of what is accepted as "right" is moving everyone in the WRONG direction if the goal is healthy, lean bodies that require little if any medical attention other than routine check-ups and trips to the "body shop" to repair the occasional bone-breaking accidents.

Body Composition

If you were going somewhere, got lost and pulled out a map, it would only be helpful if you could establish some point of reference as to where you currently are.

Knowing your composition numbers such as how much fat, water, and bone density you are carrying, tells you where you are body-wise and supplies the information you need to map out the most effective way to get to your desired destination, "Leandom."

A traditional scale simply cannot, does not, will not provide the most important aspect of your total weight, which is the percentage of body fat you are currently carrying.

When you measure your body-fat percentage, you are determining what percentage of your total body weight is fat and how much is lean body mass (muscles, bones and organs) and water. TurboChargers strive to preserve and enhance their lean body mass while minimizing their excess internal and external body fat.

Bottom line: Diet claims based on success in pounds should be ignored if body fat has not been accurately measured.

Body fat is all you want to lose! "Weight loss" is just a lower number on the scale that comes along for the ride.

Today, most bodies carry about 25% body fat for men, 35% for women. Certainly many bodies register considerably higher. At these measurements or higher, the body is obese, and chronic degenerative disease is building or already present. Healthful body-fat percentages for men begin at about 15% and about 22% for women. These percentages will likely improve health and move you into a lower risk for disease. However, the lower your body-fat percentage, *within the acceptable ranges*, the healthier you will become. TurboCharged men who really seek to reach ultimate levels of lean aim for a body-fat percentage in the 8-12% range and women aim for 13.5-18% (up to 22% for women who desire to become pregnant).

Once you have a way to measure body fat, you will finally be able to track the loss of the only thing you want to lose, **body fat**. You don't get healthier by fasting or going on a rapid-weight-loss program if what you are losing is muscle, bone, water or any other essential body component.

A Free Body-Fat Calculator

As we stated right up front: There is NOTHING special you must buy to be a TurboCharger.

Believe it or not, the most accurate body-fat measurement reference we have found (thanks to our friend "The Admiral") is the US Navy calculator, which uses only two measurements for men and three for women along with your height. Log on to www.turbocharged.us.com to get a reading of your current body composition right now.

Studies document that there is a direct relationship between neck and waist measurements when calculating body fat. All things being equal, the greater the difference between the two, the lower the body fat. If your neck stays the same and your waist measurement goes down, you are losing excess fat. That's what is supposed to happen. However, if you have some fat on your neck, that measurement will decrease. Hopefully, a lot less than your waist measurement!

We have also found with men that each 1" decrease in waist measurement equals about a five-to-seven pound reduction in weight. The greater your actual fat loss, the greater the waist-measurement reduction.

Right now there is nothing preventing you from truly measuring success for the first time in your dieting history. Get your tape measure out. Take the measurements of your height, neck and abdomen for men and also hips for women. Load the numbers into your computer and within seconds you will get a reading of your body-fat percentage. When you use this, we have only one word of advice: Make sure you load your information under the correct sex (male or female) column or your results will be highly inaccurate!

If you want to get detailed day-to-day measurements, you can invest in a home-use body-fat scale. A cheap body-fat scale will cost around $30 and an expensive one about $200. Tanita makes a very good one starting at about $99. (Note: We have no affiliation with Tanita. It just happens to be a good brand.) Whichever brand you choose, a scale that measures both weight and body-fat percentage will give you far more accurate information about your body and health than the old traditional scale you've been using.

The cheaper scales may not be as sensitive, so it might take two or three days to see the body fat that you will lose as you become TurboCharged. The better scales will give you a good daily reading, while tracking your muscle mass, bone mass, water percentage, bio-metabolic age vs. calendar age, and even more information depending on the model. You can get one at a sporting goods store or search online. They are easy to use and customized to the user. They are not perfect, but the difference in what you will learn is night and day compared to basic weight scales.

A home-use body-fat scale won't match exactly with the Navy calculator. There is an inaccuracy with all these types of body-fat measurements that is generally about 4% +/- variation. The only real way to measure body fat accurately is the three or four "compartment" model, which is a very expensive lab procedure. Even more accurate is to be a cadaver and have the fat extracted and weighed...but clearly this isn't a viable option!

In the morning when everyone is dehydrated, body fat will read higher by about 2-5 percent. This is normal. An hour or so after sufficient hydration has occurred, body-fat readings will drop. Although body-fat scales provide the most accurate readings two or three hours after eating or drinking in the late morning or early afternoon, we realize it is probably not convenient for most TurboChargers to get naked and weigh yourself in the middle of the day.

Taking this into consideration, consistency with the time you weigh-in will provide the best data. Know that if you consistently weigh yourself every morning upon awakening, the numbers will ultimately result in a pattern. This will not be your most accurate reading because you are dehydrated after a long night's sleep and you may be getting ready for "elimination" that could change your weight by as much as a pound. The important thing is to simply get on your scale every day at the same time. Use the chart it comes with or download one from our site www.TurboCharged.us.com. You will immediately be able to track your daily progress.

Besides measuring your body fat…use a mirror. Visual changes will be apparent quite quickly as you TurboCharge. Carefully watch both muscle and belly appearance and you will be delightfully surprised and inspired to stay on track.

Ideal Body Weight and Body-Fat Calculation Variations

Although some medical organizations will tell you that the weights in the Metropolitan Life Insurance chart below are best suited for younger people, we strongly disagree. We, your authors, at first printing of this book, are right at the edge of 50 or mid-50s. Individually, we weigh-in at the lower numbers shown for "ideal weight" in relation to our heights. Our body-fat percentages are at the lower end of the healthful range when we weigh-in on either our Tanita scales or when using the Naval calculator.

Don't pick a "weight" goal. Weight goals serve as a guideline but won't give you essential information. Instead, focus on body fat as a percentage of your overall weight. For men, 8-15% body fat is lean and will make you very happy. If you are a female, with 13.5-22% body fat you will be quite slender and very shapely. Always choose a body-fat goal and never accept "losing weight" as a goal or your brain will oblige you and drop muscle, too. If you choose to eat non-turbocharged foods, pay attention to any increase in your body fat. If your body fat shows increases of 1-2% for more than a day or two, focus on eating TurboCharged foods only, until you are back into your healthy and lean safety zone. You will be able to do this much more easily than you think or have been able to do on other programs in the past because of your new high-fat burning metabolism.

Men Ideal Weight	Height	Women Ideal Weight
	4'11"	95
	5'0"	100
	5'1"	105
118	5'2"	110
124	5'3"	115
130	5'4"	120
136	5'5"	125
142	5'6"	130
148	5'7"	135
154	5'8"	140
160	5'9"	145
166	5'10"	150
172	5'11"	155
178	6'0"	160

184	6'1"
190	6'2"
196	6'3"
202	6'4"

Now that you know how to measure fat, the only thing that will accurately determine and document your success, let's learn a bit about a true, totally natural and free fat-burning elixir.

Step #3
The Fat-Burning Elixir

U nless you are TurboCharged, most likely you are in the habit of eating until you are full. TurboChargers know how to help their bodies feel full so they can rapidly get to their destination: a lean, shapely and healthy teenage figure. And yes, that is your realistic goal! Right now you will learn another simple step. In less than 72 hours, this step will allow you to retrain your appetite to be very satisfied with less food. Food that is nutritionally potent will satisfy you and will make you feel really, really good. We promise.

Hunger vs. Appetite

There is a big difference between hunger and appetite. Hunger is the cry that a newborn child experiences and lets the whole house know. As a parent, you soon learn to distinguish the hunger cry versus the lonely, angry or simply baby cries. Hunger is an instinctive signal that declares the body's need for food.

Appetite is altogether different. Appetite is a memory. You can recognize it when you feel a desire for a specific food, like burgers and fries or pizza and a soda. Appetite is the mechanism whereby your brain stores your likes and dislikes of certain foods. If you crave something specific, always be aware it is probably appetite calling, not hunger. The one exception may be the cravings of a pregnant woman. Such cravings may be calling for necessary nutrients.

What you also may not realize is that there is also a big difference between hunger and thirst. According to many anthropologists, our primitive instincts of thirst are far stronger than our instincts of hunger. Yet most of us often confuse thirst for hunger. Prior to this book, you likely have not read that confusing thirst for hunger may be a major contributor to obesity. As you learn how to TurboCharge your body, you will be learning to use new tools to help you recognize the difference between hunger and thirst.

For starters, let us tell you now: If you walk around sipping from a water bottle all day you are not yet TurboCharged.

Thirst vs. Hunger

Did you know that it becomes very difficult to survive more than about three days without water? Yet it has been proven that people can live over 40 days without food before causing serious damage to their bodies. More often than not, when we think we are hungry, what we really are is thirsty.

Thirst is often not experienced before a level of 4-5% dehydration is reached, but at 2% dehydration, "hunger" signals from your brain are usually triggered, and this effect increases as we age.

So again, what is simply dehydration is often perceived as hunger.

When you learn to recognize your true thirst instinctively, you will begin simultaneously and automatically to reduce your food intake. Just as if you think you are hungry when you are more likely thirsty, when you have eaten and then feel thirsty, your body is giving you the clue you need to stop eating food and start drinking. Keep this in mind if you are drinking alcohol with a meal. As you notice your thirst begin to rise toward the end of a meal, it is water your body is calling for, not another sip of wine or an alcohol-based cocktail.

We will talk about exercise later, but for now, suffice it to say that strenuous exercise will usually make this thirst/hunger confusion worse. What the body needs after exercise is rehydration, with water being the single best option. However, too often our tendency is to reach for food or a so-called nutrition bar that is loaded with fat and carbohydrates, or perhaps drink some sugar-laden sports concoction that results in consuming more calories than we need. Making incorrect food choices can actually result in even greater dehydration.

Most plant foods (except nuts and grains) are composed of about 85-90% water. This may be the reason dehydration triggers hunger, because eating plant foods would have nurtured and rehydrated our ancestors, according to medical anthropologist Mark Davis. Even raw animal foods are fairly high in moisture content, about 70% water. Davis theorized that selective pressures during our evolution may have efficiently consolidated the mechanisms signaling hunger and thirst.

A sufficient water intake (we call it "filling your tank") has a profound effect on physiology since it lowers the body's response to sugar ingested, improves insulin sensitivity and promotes fat burning for energy.

Conversely, dehydration results in inhibited fat burning and lean-tissue loss, while contributing to all sorts of metabolic problems, along with increased moodiness.

Water does so many good things that it is hard to overemphasize its value. Adequate water intake:

◦ Raises testosterone levels, improving muscle maintenance and fat burning;

◦ Increases your metabolism, causing body fat to be utilized instead of lean mass;

◦ Lubricates joints and can eliminate many bone and joint problems, including arthritis;

◦ Creates super-immunity and eliminates allergies, colds and flu. The body cannot fight off diseases if it is burdened with waste. The mucous membranes and cells must be constantly flushed with water to allow toxins and waste to be quickly removed, allowing natural defenses to kill foreign bodies such as harmful bacteria. No one need ever get a cold or flu again!

And…as a last but not least TurboCharged advantage…

◦ In sufficient quantity, water fills the stomach, stretching it so we feel full and our satiety hormones are released. Right now, it probably takes way too much food to trigger this response, which consequently results in more overeating. This is because your stomach size has likely doubled over the years as a result of too many big dinners. Water, in sufficient quantity, eliminates false hunger and unnecessary eating.

What TurboChargers Know About Surgery, Tight Belts and Water

Let's take a little walk down memory lane and throw a bit of science into the picture as well. At one time or another, you've probably read about some seriously obese celebrity who decided to lose their excess body fat by going under the scalpel for what we believe is unnecessary and dangerous bariatric surgery or "laparoscopic" stomach banding.

The rationale behind this surgery rests on the fact that the stomach capacity of overweight individuals is almost double that of lean subjects. When gastric balloons are inserted into stomachs, filling 2/3 of capacity, appetite is significantly reduced. Why? Simply, fullness is achieved with gastric balloons, causing far more appetite suppression as satiety hormones are more readily released and recognized. The weight loss that occurs after laparoscopic banding surgery for the very obese is not influenced by less glucose or hormonal differences. Rather, the weight loss is due to the fact that the stomach is smaller in size as a result of the banding, so less food fits. The research behind this surgery concludes that the sensation of a full gut resulted in cessation of appetite and greater satiety (read that as satisfaction from foods eaten with less subsequent hunger) for extended periods, which in turn leads to the reduction of excessive food intake.

To imagine the effect of a "belted bariatric surgery," picture this: Recall one of those big dinners when your body gave you plenty of cues to stop eating. Remember too, that instead of listening, you simply decided to loosen your belt a notch or two? A tight belt around your waistline imitates this bariatric effect. The "tightness" and limited expansion ability causes important hormones to be released, telling the brain to cease sending hunger signals. A tight belt or a stomach topped off with plenty of water following a meal will simulate this same effect…much more safely than surgery.

This little science lesson explains why we TurboChargers don't walk around sipping from a water bottle. Do you think this idea of drinking lots of water or keeping a belt tight is crazy? Laugh at this simple wisdom all you want or choose to listen and get TurboCharged.

TurboChargers Don't Sip Water, We Fill Our Tanks!

Water delivers the "viscosity" your engine requires. Water literally keeps you "fluid" in every sense of the word. A little-known fact is that refined foods and the resulting high insulin levels eliminate thirst. This means most people are in a constant and dangerous state of dehydration and they don't know it. The next time you are very thirsty, eat something like chocolate or a meal high in fat and carbohydrate. Your thirst magically disappears but your dehydration level is increasing. (BTW, drinking alcohol has the same effect so don't use it as a fluid substitute.) Dehydration stops the flow of natural cleansing, resulting in sticky mucous that in turn makes the body more vulnerable to sickness and general lack of energy. Higher insulin levels cause the body to retain water as opposed to the "flushing" that is so necessary for dead cells to be removed along with undesired bacteria. Salt also causes the body to retain water, but less so than sugar and other meals that result in higher insulin levels. When you are new to TurboCharging and are actively seeking to reduce your body fat rapidly, maximum hydration, primarily with water, and secondarily with other zero-calorie drinks, is essential to triggering the release of hormones that results in the sensation of satiety or satisfaction with lower food intake. This step gives your brain the signal that you are satisfied and full. As you reach TurboCharged status and all of your natural bodily functions are working synergistically in high gear, you can reduce the level of fluid intake because your TurboCharged foods are naturally high in moisture. Your brain will also be functioning to receive satiety signals that preserve your new-found leanness.

Sipping water will not help you to TurboCharge your body. If you want to experience the natural fabulosity of a lean and healthy body, ignore the advice of nutritionists and other such gurus who tell you to carry a water bottle around with you. While regular sips of water may keep you hydrated, if you want to reduce your hunger and get lean, the true value of water while dieting involves filling and stretching your stomach. TurboChargers know we must create the sensation of a full and satisfied belly: a full belly that feels comparable to the fullness we may have experienced from those big Thanksgiving meals and other gustatory celebrations.

Instead of eating more food, we TurboChargers fill our tanks with plenty of water.

Feelings of hunger can usually be eliminated entirely by following this TurboCharged step. Putting this into practice is wildly easy:

- Drink 2-3 glasses of water (16-32 ounces) upon awakening or ideally 1-2 quarts of water within the first two hours of rising each day and fill your tank again when hungry.

- Before any meal and immediately after, drink up. Aim for at least 16 ounces, and closer to 32 ounces. Drink water until you feel full.

🍶 The minute you notice thirst while eating a meal, stop eating and drink up. Your body has sent you a message.

By consuming up to two quarts of water immediately upon feeling hungry, you will be stretching your stomach, which will release satiety hormones, increase metabolism, speed body-fat release, retain muscle, improve skin tone and cleanse your body. TurboChargers live by this vital step. This step is extremely healthy, raises immunity substantially and greatly aids in the processing of your body fat.

Make sure you fill your tank with 16-32 ounces of water first thing in the morning, because whenever you are dehydrated, you will think you are hungry even though what you need is water. We are usually dehydrated before we ever receive the first thirst signals. Keep this foremost in your mind and you absolutely, positively will succeed in TurboCharging your body! Simple, right? Drink as much water as you need to feel full. In the evening, feel free to slow down your drinking so you aren't being awakened throughout the night by "nature's call."

Being properly hydrated, as we have just explained, is an extremely simple yet breakthrough fat-loss and health secret. The sheer volume of non-caloric fluid, ideally water, coupled with the TurboCharged foods you will learn about in Step #7 will trigger other satiety hormones as well. This easy-to-implement step completely eliminates hunger, sometimes for many hours. So set times in your day, no more than two or three hours apart, to "fill up" with water. Also, remember to fill up as soon as you feel any pangs of hunger or if, during or after a meal, you notice you are thirsty or your mouth becomes dry. Repeat this step by drinking up, and the appetite suppression will continue.

Alcohol, Caffeine, Teas, Diet Sodas and TurboCharging

Alcohol

Since alcohol is a liquid, let's talk a minute about drinking it. You can drink alcohol when TurboCharging, but you must limit consumption.

Hard alcohol and wine can cause both loss of muscle mass and dehydration. More than a glass or two of wine or one shot of hard alcohol could cause a crash (literally) or set you back. Alcohol is dehydrating. Sometimes people unintentionally keep drinking alcohol to excess because they don't realize it is increasing their thirst. So if you are going to have a martini or a glass of wine, make sure you are also drinking plenty of water at the same time. The water will keep you hydrated and counter the tendency of alcohol to test willpower. Finally, and this is VERY IMPORTANT: Keep in mind that TurboCharging makes your body much more efficient at processing anything. Therefore any alcohol is likely to "get to your head" much more quickly with a lot less consumption than you may be used to. Be extra careful with alcohol consumption if you need to drive or operate any machinery. Your entire body is becoming more efficient and this includes how quickly it will process alcohol of any kind. Also, watch your mixes. Seltzer water and club soda are the only mixers we recommend, besides water or ice! Our best advice would be to keep alcohol consumption to no more than one drink a day and preferably not more than three times a week when you want to lose body fat rapidly.

Coffee

Coffee, or more specifically, caffeine in itself, is an interesting study. As far as we can determine, 50% of the research supports caffeine consumption and 50% cites detrimental effects. "Pro" studies suggest that coffee improves fat burning by mobilizing fat stores. In our experience there is no difference with or without it. Some use coffee or tea and creamer (or sugar-free whey protein) as a meal, and they claim it quickly eliminates their appetite on this program. However, too much caffeine can cause jitters and can create mood swings and insulin spikes. This can lead to an unnecessary detour as you try to calm your frazzled nerves. We recommend no more than two cups a day. If you are using any kind of creamer, it should be no more than two tablespoons of half-and-half. Not fat-free, skim, 1 or 2%, whole milk, sweetened soy, almond, coconut or anything else, all of which would be either too high in sugar and/or unnecessary additives. And absolutely don't use chemical, processed creamers either. P.S.: Watch out for those Starbucks (and other coffee chain) large coffees with all the syrups. These are 100% fat-building drinks. We will explain why in Step #7.

Tea

Tea, especially green tea, may have health and fat-burning properties, but they are not easily demonstrated or readily apparent. All green teas and most regular teas have antioxidants and other beneficial properties that are great, but we are already consuming many antioxidants with TurboCharged foods. Antioxidants are beneficial, but nothing comes closer to stimulating antioxidants than the very low calorie levels of this plan and nothing has more naturally occurring antioxidants than fruits and vegetables in general. Any high-caffeine tea will affect your body as coffee does. Some people are more sensitive to caffeine and become jittery so drink it based on your enjoyment and reaction, while limiting yourself to two caffeinated cups of anything per day. When we speak of other noncaloric fluids, we recommend you select from mint, chamomile, lemongrass, ginger or other naturally occurring caffeine-free options, when you seek more variety. Another favorite is simply a cinnamon stick in hot water. And, be careful about adding anything to your coffee or tea. No honey, agave nectar or sugar of any kind. Any of these will shut down your TurboCharger.

Diet Sodas and Soft Drinks

Diet drinks are unrestricted, but we aren't going to tell you they will support your long-term health. There is evidence that carbonated water depletes minerals, so non-carbonated drinks or ice water are better. Further, artificially sweetened sodas and beverages can sometimes increase hunger, so water or naturally caffeine-free tea is better. If you insist on your diet sodas, try to limit them to no more than two a day.

When Hunger is Thirst

Dave Curtis, age 56, is a busy CFO of a high-technology company. At 5'10", his average adult weight was 186.5 pounds with 25% body fat. After four months of TurboCharging, he weighed 161.5 pounds with 16% body fat, and now has a 31-inch waistline.

"At my age, this is just remarkable," says Dave. "I must confess I do not work the program perfectly. I enjoy the occasional glass of wine and mix meat and vegetables in greater quantities than suggested, but it still works great."

What Dave does follow explicitly is the TurboCharged step for drinking water. He learned firsthand that thirst often masquerades as hunger. "I drink four eight-ounce glasses of water every morning, and that takes away most of my appetite for a good part of the day," says Dave. "I find that when I'm sufficiently hydrated I'm far less likely to be hungry. I also find that eating foods with the complex flavors from fat, sugar and salt stimulates my appetite. Separating the food groups and eating vegetables with vegetables, fruits with fruits, and proteins with proteins, are ideal ways to really taste your food—and control your appetite."

"The eight steps, with the simple short workouts that take no time at all, are perfect for me," Dave adds. "Most of the programs I've tried over the years were way too much trouble and way too restrictive for real life. I truly believe this simple, logical and effective program is the answer to the health challenge of obesity that is rapidly, excuse the expression, *spreading* around the entire world."

Step #4
Fresh Breath Never Tasted So Good

Step #4 is short and sweet…but very important, so don't even think of skipping it. Every step of TurboCharged is remarkably simple, yet they all must be implemented in their entirety as recommended to achieve your fat-loss goal.

Here is the simple step: If you are feeling hungry, before eating anything, and before or after drinking a big glass or two of water…you need to grab some toothpaste or mouthwash, with sorbitol as one of the ingredients, and give yourself a good teeth-brushing if possible and/or swish with mouthwash. If neither toothpaste nor mouthwash are available, suck on a minty-type dissolvable strip. If possible, don't rinse, just spit. Leave a little bit of the flavor in your mouth.

Each step of TurboCharged is designed to help you work through the natural reaction of your senses to food. Each of us has countless memories stored up that associate eating food with pleasure and comfort. Food-related memories can enter the mind at any time for any reason. All five senses can stimulate the urge to eat. We see food and visualize what it will taste like. We smell food and we begin salivating. We take a little taste, our tongue perks up and we want more. We talk about food and begin recalling how something might taste. We touch food and begin thinking about how we are going to prepare a meal for consumption.

Even if we have plenty of body fat to lose or we have recently eaten, if we stimulate any of our senses with the sight, smell, taste, touch or even the thought of food, our appetite will begin to call.

When the stomach is empty, these memories can overwhelm even the most dedicated dieter. TurboChargers, however, know that this simple step, along with drinking a large quantity of water as discussed in Step #3, will immediately enable you to accelerate quickly past the memory and keep you focused on the reward—a sleek, healthy body.

This step has three noteworthy benefits:

1. It will help dull your taste buds and deaden your appetite unless you are truly hungry.

2. The miniscule bit of residual sugar or artificial sweetener in the toothpaste, mouthwash or breath strip that will remain in your mouth—after spitting but not rinsing—will send a subtle message to your brain that sugar is still plentiful. Your body recognizes this slight sugar ingestion as a good sign, so no defensive starvation action, like holding onto excess fat, is triggered.

3. If you are really hungry, this will delay a meal while you work the other steps because we all know food tastes pretty bad immediately after brushing or rinsing!

Lastly, this simple step helps get your thinking back in line. It helps get you refocused, and is of great assistance in eliminating mindless eating.

All in the TurboCharged Family

Of course we've involved our families in our pursuit of fat reduction and healthy lifestyles. Tom's sister-in-law, Julia Vogelle, 49, tried TurboCharged around the same time as she began to experience her first symptoms of menopause. Julia is an elementary school art teacher and she's incorporated the program into her life in interesting and productive ways.

"TurboCharging makes me feel great," says Julia. "I use each step several times during my day and after eating my meals. It's almost like I can feel my food turning into muscle. It's terrific. I keep my weights in a storage room by my classroom to do my exercises for about five to ten minutes at a time. Whenever my students see me exercising, they want to join in."

Julia at almost 5'8" tall, weighed 156 pounds when she decided to try TurboCharged, but had never calculated her starting percentage of body fat. In two months she weighed in at 129, with 31% body fat. She opted to ignore her calorie consumption and just work on following all the TurboCharged steps. She stopped eating all processed foods and followed the recommended food group guidelines.

"The most immediate benefit was that my menopause symptoms disappeared. No more night sweats. No more bloating and sleep interruptions. Now I sleep great and my energy level is fabulous," says Julia. "This program has given me a new understanding of my body and how it works most efficiently."

She imagines a goal weight of about 129 but she's confident that her body will find its best body-fat percentage level. "Life on the TurboCharged program is like driving my car into the automatic car wash—it comes out on the other side looking brand new." says Julia. "That's how I feel about my body. Thanks to TurboCharged, a new, healthier me has emerged."

Now let's look at how you are going to TurboCharge your fat-burning metabolism—with activity, not exercise!

Step #5
TurboCharge Your Fat-Burning Metabolism with Activity

As we stated earlier, TurboChargers focus on a reduction of their percentage of body fat instead of the number of pounds lost.

We would now like to share with you what may be another startling revelation: TurboChargers know that aerobics and bodybuilding muscle workouts actually *slow down* the time and speed it will take to reach their body-fat reduction goals. Shocked? You should be, considering that every major "weight loss expert" and health institution has been saying for years that to achieve and maintain weight loss you must do 30 to 90 minutes of aerobic exercise three to five times a week along with several strength training sessions. Who has the time or the desire? They recommend that you cut calories and work out vigorously for an hour on average every day. Sounds like a prescription for major grumpiness and an urge to binge!

Stating the obvious: Obesity is rampant. The problem, in our estimation, is that most people are approaching health and weight loss in the same way we approach our day jobs: We cut out the good stuff while making exercise "work," using clinical, repetitious and supposedly scientific maneuvers while we forget about the fun we could be having if we simply became active.

TurboCharged is not an anti-exercise program. Exercise is great for your cardiovascular health and general well-being. However, TurboChargers know that long or strenuous exercise is simply not a requirement for losing body fat, and further, that it can actually be counterproductive and slow down progress if calories are reduced or not high enough to compensate for the energy expended. TurboChargers get lean first by following all eight steps, including incorporating more activity wherever possible. After we are TurboCharged and lean, if we want to train for a marathon or a hike up Mt. Kilimanjaro, we can do it!

More Activity is the Goal

Activity is essential for a healthy body and spirit. Activity is what you need when you are in the process of eliminating excess body fat. Please reread those two sentences. TurboChargers purposely do not use the word "exercise." Instead, TurboChargers, when they are in the process of getting lean, get moving and work on being more active. Once they have reached their ideal body-fat percentage, they do whatever activities or exercises their hearts desire. (No pun intended!)

Activity is what will make the difference between health and illness. It is a natural stress reliever and good for overall health and maintenance of a sleek and youthful body. Unless your current circumstances or your doctor prohibit you from moving, get out and get active!

Regular activity is much better than "exercising when you have the time." Regular activity is equally important to your physical health and your mental well-being.

The activity recommended in the TurboCharged program will not increase your hunger, but high levels of aerobics and all strenuous exercise will. Please reread that last sentence again, too.

A Science Lesson on Calculating Your Energy Requirements

A calorie represents the specific amount of energy in the form of heat created by your body "burning up" any particular amount of food you opt to eat or the amount of energy burned up by your body to perform any activity. We are always in need of calories as we are always burning them for energy. This said, if you consume more calories in a day than you burn up, your excess calories get stored as body fat. Average people burn about 15 calories per pound of body weight (your weight x 15 = calories necessary to maintain your current weight). Teenage boys typically need about 20 calories per pound of body weight, whereas teen girls need closer to 17. Active people need more calories. For example, swimming burns 400-675 calories in an hour. A fast walk burns 330 calories in an hour. On the flipside, TV watching or Internet surfing burns only 40 calories an hour. Let's delve more into this "activity" picture.

How activity levels have changed...

Our early ancestors likely spent their days seeking food, water, safety and shelter. Big leisurely meals as we know them today were highly unlikely. Our ancestors were energetic. If they weren't sleeping, they were always up and actively doing something.

Early farmers using a horse-drawn plow likely used up to 600 calories an hour to cultivate their crops. Today, a farmer driving a tractor with a steering wheel needs only 170 calories an hour. Add power steering and that number is down to only 136 calories an hour. Today, they can even eat and plow at the same time.

Household chores once required about 250 calories per hour. Today, considering all the appliances being used in the average household (including robotic vacuums), the number is down to about 120 calories an hour or less.

Television is adding more fat to our bodies than perhaps any other invention with the exception of the automobile. Isn't this ironic when you think about the incessant barrage of advertisements on TV that promote new ways to lose weight and shape up? Isn't it funny that none ever suggest turning off the old telly, getting up, and taking a walk, or even a nap for that matter! Estimates reveal the majority of us spend as much as a third of our waking hours simply staring at a television set. That equals two to four hours daily. Imagine what you could be doing with that time! For example, you could have gone out dancing for an hour, chatted it up with friends sitting and talking for another two hours and burned a likely total of about 408 calories (depending on what kind of dancer you are!). Plus, you'd probably have a lot more fun.

Let's look at something as simple as the evolution of the early typewriter compared to computer keyboards of today. A typist using a standard mechanical typewriter needed strength! If you are our age, you remember having to pound those keys! A secretary likely expended about 88 calories an hour while sitting and typing. The arrival of electronic typewriters brought this caloric expenditure down to about 73 calories an hour. This difference of 15 calories an hour or 105 calories in a seven-hour workday, times a five-day workweek, is a reduction of 525 calories a week. In about a year, this secretary would gain about six pounds if she kept her eating and all other activity at the same prior levels. Add the "texting" component and brevity of emails today and calorie (energy) requirements are virtually nonexistent.

If when traveling to a destination 2.5 miles away, you choose to walk, you could easily be there in an hour walking at a moderately brisk pace and you'd use up 210 calories. If you chose to ride your bicycle, you would likely be there in about 27 minutes and you'd have expended 122 calories. Yet using the option to drive, although you will arrive at your destination in about six minutes, you will have burned only 17 calories.

Unless you are an active construction worker or "high-voltage guy" (like our brother who climbs utility poles all day), or unless you are TurboCharged, your lack of activity is making you lethargic and sick while eroding your muscle and adding lots of fat.

As you can see, although technological advances are wonderful in many ways, these developments have been detrimental to our health in countless ways because thanks (or no thanks) to them, our activity levels have dramatically decreased. What we are addressing in these pages is the fact that we have gotten fatter as the amount of our daily activity has decreased.

The Problem with Exercise

The exercise conundrum is three-fold as we see it:

1) Exercise for exercise's sake alone just doesn't fit our lifestyles. It is not fun, it can be boring, and many of us simply lack the time or inclination to do it.

2) Thirty to ninety minutes of daily exercise while cutting calories, makes it very hard not to crave the very food you are trying so hard to eliminate.

3) If you sit at a desk, TV or computer for most of the day, even if you exercise 45 minutes four to five times a week, you are still a couch potato.

While you are in the initial process of TurboCharging, when you are leaning out your body, bringing your body-fat percentage down to its ideal high-performance levels, the only "exercise" your body requires is the good old kind of activity you'll see in the list on page 44 along with a few short walks during the day and the three to five minutes of daily muscle power routines we will discuss in Step #6.

So please listen up! You can TurboCharge your body even if you are bed-ridden. Yes—you read that right. You can get all the way down to a sleeker, healthier body with the minimal activity that we outline in *TurboCharged*. Tom recently had a significant knee operation. Yet in the many subsequent recovery weeks, he actually maintained most of his muscle, while remaining lean and fabulous.

Please take some time to carefully review the list of activities in the pages ahead. TurboChargers make activity a daily part of life. You don't have to "get to it" as in "getting to the gym." TurboChargers incorporate simple activity. You opt to walk up a flight of stairs instead of taking the elevator. You take a morning, after-lunch or post-dinner stroll. You take your dog for a walk. You add a hill or stairs, and you TurboCharge your fat-burning leg muscles because you must also lift your entire body weight against the force of gravity, which calls for extra effort and the increased expenditure of energy, which means more fat burned. For each mile, which can be accomplished in a briskly paced 15 minutes, you will burn about 122 calories almost exclusively from fat, and your leg muscles will strengthen and build, which in turn will ultimately cause more calories to burn.

Activity, to be effective, does not have to leave you breathless and perspiring. Extended strenuous activity is not necessary to keep body fat under control. A moderate and consistent increase in your daily activity, day after day, is much more effective than random spurts on a weekend. Minutes of activity each day ultimately add up over a week. These additional energy expenditures and other benefits will add up to the loss of pounds of fat along with the strengthening and toning of lean muscle tissue. The more you are up on those legs, no matter what the activity, the need for energy triples! So get up and get TurboCharged.

Let's look at everyday activities TurboChargers do (sometimes instead of hiring someone to do it for them!). Each one helps get our bodies back on track while accessing energy requirements from stored body fat.

TurboCharge Doing Normal Stuff and Having Fun!

We provide the following list with "caloric burn" numbers because so many people are always counting their "calories burned" on the elliptical trainer, treadmill or some other aerobic exercise. Think of these numbers as a frame of reference that allows you to see that basic, everyday activities are just as effective as going to the gym, and probably much more rewarding because the activity will deliver better scenery, a cleaner house and crisp, folded laundry too!

Each activity lists a number that represents the calories burned by that activity in one minute. Multiply this number by the number of minutes being active and you'll know what you're burning as you continue to TurboCharge.

Resting, Standing & Walking

Calories Burned Per Minute

Resting in Bed	1.2
Sitting	1.4
Sitting Reading	1.4
Sitting Eating	1.6
Sitting, Playing Cards	1.7
Standing	2.8
Kneeling	1.4
Squatting	2.2
Walking Around Your House	3.4
Walking Outdoors	6.1
Walking Down Stairs	7.6
Walking Up Stairs	20.
Showering-Standing	3.7

Working Around the House

Washing Clothes	2.9
Hanging Laundry	4.7
Carrying Laundry	3.2
Sewing with Machine	1.5
Ironing Clothes	4.2
Making Beds	5.3
Mopping Floors	5.3
Sweeping Floors	1.7
Scrubbing Floors	6.0
Shaking Carpets	6.4
Peeling Vegetables	2.9
Stirring, Mixed Foods	3.0

Do It Yourself

Sawing Wood	6.9
Gardening	4.0
Carrying Tools	3.6
Shoveling	7.1
Pushing Wheelbarrow	5.2
Chopping Wood	4.9
Stacking Wood	6.1
Drilling	7.0

Sports & Hobbies

Football	10.1
Basketball	8.6
Ping Pong	4.8
Racquetball	6.0 (beginners)
Swimming	12.1
Golfing–no cart	5.5
Tennis	7.0
Bowling	8.1
Badminton	2.8
Rowing	8.0
Sailing	2.6
Playing Pool	3.0
Dancing	4.0
Horseback Riding	3.0
Cycling	8.0
Hiking	5.3
Skating-ice or roller	6.9
Skateboarding	4.0 (unless you are Tony Hawk!)
Skiing/Boarding	6.6 (unless you are Shawn White!)
Yoga	5-12 (depending on type)

And if you happen to live in Alaska, parts of Canada or anywhere else that it snows often...

Making snow angels for 20 minutes will burn 85 calories
Sleigh riding for two hours will burn 902 calories (if you walk back up that hill!)
A 30-minute snowball fight will burn 161 calories (even if you never make contact!)
An hour of snow shoveling will burn 451 calories
An hour building a snowman burns about 285 calories
Spending 30 minutes gathering logs and twigs for a fire burns about 258 calories

Walking: The TurboCharged Secret Weapon

Several studies have shown that the primary difference between overweight/obese people and lean people involves the time spent up on their feet walking versus the time spent sitting around. Walking favorably alters cholesterol, blood sugar, insulin, triglycerides and blood pressure. It increases the amount of blood pumped by the heart and therefore increases the amount of oxygen reaching all bodily tissues no matter how young, old or sedentary the person taking that walk might otherwise be. In study after study, lean people, regardless of diet, exercise or other factors, are shown to be up and moving more every day.

More than any other body part, it is our legs and butt muscles that drive our metabolism. Walking is vitally important to the resurgence of these muscles. Walking adds to your life and is fun and relaxing. More important, walking will move your metabolism into TurboCharged mode as energy is taken from body fat at a rate of 80%+. Walking also keeps appetite in abeyance. Plus, it becomes a valuable time filler, because walking everywhere possible means less time on our derrières driving our cars, watching TV, in front of a computer surfing the Internet, working at a desk or yes, eating.

Although many complain that they "don't have the time" to walk, TurboChargers consider this a poor excuse. Think of how you could add walking into your routine: using the stairs, walking up "the hill," parking farther away in the parking lot, a digestive stroll after dinner, a walk to work or to a lunch meeting, are just a few ideas. A mere 20-minute walk first thing in the morning, after lunch and again after dinner, is a very simple way to add an hour of walking to your day. Grab a friend for some conversation or meditate as you walk and take some time to observe your surroundings.

To maintain your best fat-burning pace, you should be able to carry on a conversation with a partner or sing a song if by yourself without losing your breath. A little sweat is fine, but if you can't keep the conversation going, you are moving yourself out of TurboCharged mode and working too hard for your current state of fitness. If the conversation or singing becomes strained, slow down and the fat-burning effect will actually be better at this stage of your progress. If you don't slow down, you will start feeding on the vital muscle you are working so hard to maintain.

It is easy for most of us to begin a walking regimen. Other than a comfortable pair of shoes, no special equipment is required. The duration is more important than the exertion put into it. Since the motion is continuous throughout your entire walk, so is the expenditure of energy. This fact alone makes walking the ultimate TurboCharged activity. Don't worry if you can't fit in a long walk during your busy day. A few short 10-minute walks will also keep you in TurboCharged fat-burning mode. This will also get you in shape for longer walks or hikes whenever the opportunity arises.

Walking distinguishes the lean and healthy people around the world. Even when the diet is not ideal, walking can become a tremendous lifesaver. Walking causes energy to be taken mostly from body fat, not muscle mass, and your muscles are being strengthened at the same time. A daily walk will greatly increase your metabolism. Small additions of activity in your day can really add up and will have a very positive effect, helping you to feel and look great. Some people disregard the immense benefits of walking. Why walk when you can jog, run or drive? TurboChargers know that walking is the best activity for getting sleek and lean. Once we reach the body-fat percentages that are ideal to our body type, we run whenever we want and we run faster than ever, reaching new levels of superior performance.

TurboCharged Walking Tips

To increase the impact of your walking routine, we make five simple recommendations:

1) Use a pedometer. We are big fans of the Omron Walking Style Pedometer. It costs about $30 and you can buy one at www.turbocharged.us.com. It can read your steps whether it is placed in your pocket or purse or clipped to your waist. It provides great info: total strides, distance and calories burned. We especially like that it differentiates between casual steps and faster-paced ones so you can get a good read on your actual activity levels. If you are up for a mini-challenge and want to burn fat more rapidly, aim to log a minimum of 3,600-4,000 steps on your pedometer within 30 minutes. No pedometer? Don't let this stop you. Pick a place that you can walk for two uninterrupted miles. See if you can walk the distance in 30 minutes or less. If you don't have the time to

walk for 30 minutes consecutively, don't fret. Keep that pedometer on and see how many steps you can accrue between rising and bedtime. If you get that number close to 10,000 steps daily, no matter how you do it, you will be TurboCharged in no time at all.

Recording your progress daily is a great motivational strategy. We think of our pedometers as the only personal trainers we need. They are gentle reminders to keep moving. Again, this is not necessary, but it can keep you on track and focused.

2) Add weight to your walk. Pack a backpack with some canned vegetables or ziplock baggies full of sand, put it on and stroll. Walk to the grocery store and carry your purchases home. Feel like a fat-loss splurge? For women, pick up a 4-20 pound weight vest, and for men, up to 30 pounds. Your heart rate will improve and so will the amount of fat burned. How do you choose the right weight for you? Limit the extra poundage to no more than 10% of your body weight. For example: If you weigh 140 pounds, limit your extra weight to no more than 14 pounds. Start light and build up to that number. Remember, any additional weight is adding extra resistance and is great for building those fat-burning tush and leg muscles.

3) Use your arms. Walking poles are another option to add your arms into the muscle-building routine of walking. Simply go the natural free route with two straight sticks right out of the woods. A *Journal of Strength and Conditioning Research* article claims that 67% more calories will be burned with walking sticks vs. basic walking thanks to the additional arm motion.

4) Walk your dog. If you have a dog, take him or her walking with you. Company can be fun. Plus, the natural tugging of the leash will add subtle stress to your arms while you walk, thereby increasing the value of this activity.

5) Try a brief sprint. If you are ready and want to really boost fat burning during a walk, try this TurboCharged technique: Walk at your normal pace for awhile to warm up, then sprint for up to one minute or until it starts to feel stressful or you become winded, whichever comes first. This TurboCharged boost will burn more calories for every minute you walk, not just those when you are sprinting. It will keep your metabolic rate high without overstressing your body, and the good news is you will continue to burn fat at a higher rate over the next few hours. Remember: The goal of a sprint is not to get into a full-out aerobic workout. The objective is simply to push a little and then resume your regular speed as you catch your breath. These short sprints will build leg strength and really help you in those times that you need to catch a bus, chase after hyperactive children or jump safely out of the way of that oncoming NYC taxi!

Note: Some people like gadgets. A heart rate monitor will help you realize you are going out of your ideal range for maximum fat burning. However, no gadgets are required for TurboCharging. Simply pay attention to your ability to converse or sing, while running or taking a little sprint. If you are having trouble catching your breath, you have stepped out of your ideal fat-burning mode. S…l…o…w… down and you will *SPEED UP* fat burning.

Activity of Any Kind Will Keep You TurboCharged

How many people cruise the parking lot in front of a store, or worse, their gym, looking for the closest spot? Ridiculous, isn't it? Start looking for ways to walk more and not less! Always be on the lookout for ways to incorporate more activity into your life. Park farther away, not closer! Squeeze your buttocks muscles while you wait for your coffee to brew and hot water to boil or do leg raises to the side and rear. Suck your stomach in tightly on the grocery store line or while sitting in traffic. Return your shopping cart to the proper spot. Do a few standing push-ups off the kitchen counter before washing dishes. Vacuum your house and bend to get under the couch. Iron your clothes and flex up and down on your tippy toes to strengthen vital leg muscles. The goal is not to become a professional athlete. Your objective is to keep moving so your entire body becomes a superior fat-burning machine. You can do it. Be creative. Then please log onto www.turbocharged.us.com and share the creative ways you are incorporating activity into your daily schedule and busy life.

Meet One Real TurboCharged Jerry Lewis

Jerry Lewis, of Tiburon, California, has heard all of the jokes you can imagine about his name. This Jerry Lewis is not the iconic comedian, nor the piano-charging country singer; however, he is a fascinating individual in his own right. A retired CEO from the mortgage benefits industry, he owns and runs a pistachio farm and is thinking of someday writing a book about his favorite nuts.

At age 69, Jerry is an avid mountain biker, kayaker and fly fisherman. He is eager to share how his experience with TurboCharged far exceeded his expectations.

Jerry weighed 192 pounds for most of his adult life. People told him he carried the weight well on his 6' frame, but he wanted to weigh less and reduce his percentage of body fat.

"Nothing worked until I heard about TurboCharged in November 2009. I followed the directions in every way," says Jerry, "including drinking so much water that I always needed to scope out the nearest bathroom, and I completely gave up the foods I learned were damaging to my success."

The process was much easier than he thought possible, and the results, to him, were amazing. "This program is not about perfection," says Jerry, "it's about achieving an intelligent balance so that you eat and move to look and feel your best and not feel deprived. That's not just the promise of TurboCharged, it's what this program actually delivers."

In 30 days, Jerry's weight dropped from 192 to 175, and his body-fat percentage decreased from 26% to 20%, which he has had no problem maintaining. "I have never been busier or more actively engaged in my life. I was high-energy before, but after TurboCharging, my wife and I agree that I'm more energized than ever," says Jerry.

Step #6
Muscle Power in 5...
Minutes a Day!

Many years ago, a researcher, Hans Selye, theorized that when humans are under any kind of stress, the brain doesn't differentiate as to whether our stress is a positive or negative experience. All activities including partying, dancing at a wedding or driving a race car, are perceived as stress by your body. Good stress, but stress nonetheless. Sitting in traffic, arguments, work and home pressure are also stressful. This is the kind of stress you want to curtail or manage. When that good or bad stress causes your heartbeat to change, defensive hormones are released and you notice you feel different. Doc Childre, in his book *The Heart Math Solution*, further studied our physical responses to stress and how these detrimentally affect our hearts and long-term health. Bottom line: Stress causes the brain to take muscle and convert it to glucose to give the body an extra jolt of blood sugar, which is harmful to our arteries. When you are dieting and exercising or living in a stressful environment, you are losing vital muscle and damaging your heart muscle at the same time.

Since all reduced-calorie diets are stressful and perceived as starvation, the brain goes into a defensive mode. It responds by converting vital lean body mass for more energy to make up the calorie deficit. If you are like most people, the odds are high that your body is getting the majority of its energy needs from a constant supply of sugar in the foods you eat.

Until you become TurboCharged and your body becomes efficient at using body fat for energy instead of sugar, in times of need, it is much easier for your body to convert some of your lean body mass (muscle) into glucose instead of using your stored fat. This is not what you want!

Traditional weight-loss diets raise a red flag to the brain as your sugar supply runs low. This is experienced as distress, anxiety and intense hunger. Your body will start to convert muscle into glucose. Your brain senses a problem. It knows that loss of muscle mass is not good. It begins sending messages to eat as it is fighting for the return of the muscle and other lean body mass that is being lost. This intense hunger continues to increase until you give in and eat. Usually you end up eating too much. As a result, lean body mass is restored—but so is added body fat as a "protector" to defend against muscle loss in the future. If you have tried traditional diets, you have probably experienced this condition firsthand. You have watched your willpower fail. Now you know why. Your brain is very powerful. To succeed you need to work with it, not against it.

If you diet without the TurboCharged steps your brain will perceive starvation and react defensively. Each step of TurboCharged works to remind our brains that nutrients are plentiful and muscle is necessary. The combination of these steps is carefully designed so there is no sense of starvation, danger or attack—which would be impossible to combat as we would be fighting against well-established, evolutionary, survival forces.

Excess Body Fat is Fuel

The purpose of Step #6 is to lead your brain to source your body fat for energy instead of your muscle or that bag of chips. Once your brain realizes there is plenty of stored fat hanging out just waiting to be consumed and your body simultaneously receives the plentiful nutrients that are in the foods you will be eating (Step #7), your body starts to cooperate and assist you in your fat-reducing goals. You are suddenly TurboCharged. The brain no longer reacts as if it is facing the stress of a dangerously restricted food supply. Gently stressing your muscles will elevate your metabolism and your brain is directed to a bountiful new food source: YOUR EXCESS BODY FAT!

A primary goal of TurboCharging is to get your body to use excess body fat as its preferred energy source. Creating positive "stress" that directs your body to burn your body fat for energy can be accomplished in just one minute. Your muscles are the best calorie-burning tissue the body has. When muscles are called into action regularly—even with a simple one-minute workout—muscles will be maintained or even increase while your fat-burning ability also increases significantly.

To begin TurboCharging, all you have to do is 3-5 cycles of Step #6 each day. Think of these as mini-muscle workouts that keep your body burning fat. Gently yet regularly you are giving your brain a nudging reminder that you need your muscles, so it must continue to draw energy requirements from fat, not muscle. The muscle you will be building with these mini-routines will be sleek and long, more like that of a basketball player, acrobat, gymnast, ballerina or healthy active teenager. You don't have to worry that you might "bulk up" as that is not the goal of TurboCharged. To bulk up, your routine would need to be long, hard and anaerobic. This would actually trigger your body to cannibalize some of your muscle for energy instead of using your body fat in addition to increasing hunger. You will be building elasticity and tone.

Simplicity in your muscle "stressing" choices will work just fine. You can achieve your goals the good old-fashioned Marine way with push-ups, pull-ups and sit-ups or any of the other mini-muscle power routines we provide here and on www.TurboCharged.us.com. Also, you don't need to rush out and buy dumbbells. Many basic household items like a can or two of vegetables from your cupboard or even a full plastic container of laundry detergent can substitute effectively.

If one day you feel like splurging and want to purchase some dumbbells, go for it. Often you can pick them up for a couple of dollars at yard sales from sellers who don't know how to get TurboCharged. If you buy dumbbells, women should pick up a hand-held starter set of 3, 5, 8 or 10 pounds maximum. Men will need a set ranging from 10 to 30 pounds. Women should start with a weight that allows them to get to 10 repetitions, working up to 15, with the last three being more stressful. For men, pick them up and use the same approach. Use a weight that allows 6-8 reps with stress but not strain, then push a little harder for a total of 10.

The goal is not to intensely "pump iron" but only to work and hold onto the muscle you already have. After a few TurboCharged weeks, if the weights start to feel light or you want to increase muscle size, the heavier the weight the better. But even then be cautious so you don't hurt yourself. The two original fitness gurus, Jack LaLanne and Paul Bragg, who both lived to their late 90s, always said that the worst fitness mistake anyone can make is trying to get in shape in a day because that approach is guaranteed to cause you pain. This hurt can take you off your mission of leanness and might also result in serious longer-term injuries.

Most of us have enough muscle. These resistance repetitions are designed to retain and shape the muscle you have and are not anaerobic. Heavy weight training, whether dieting or not, will make you hungry, cause you to overeat and make losing body fat much more difficult. All strenuous exercise using heavy weight is too stressful and is counterproductive during a fat-loss program. The same is true of aerobic-type exercise, as we will repeat throughout this book. If you continue to follow each TurboCharged step you will find that these mini-routines will not make you as hungry as traditional exercise will. In fact, they may eliminate hunger!

If you are like us and have spent hundreds or even thousands of dollars on gym memberships, home equipment and all the accoutrements that are constantly being hawked on television as necessary or required for getting in shape...let us assure you unequivocally that this is unnecessary. Those days are over if you want them to be over. You do not need special clothes, trips to the gym, expensive machines or anything more than your own body weight and determination to reach your goal of a TurboCharged body.

Once you really understand and are working the program, feel free to expand your one-minute routines to two and then perhaps three minutes every two to three hours throughout the day, or whenever you feel hungry. Seriously, this really is the maximum you will ever need to look amazing, whether you are a man or a woman.

TurboCharged in One Minute

Whenever you feel hunger, fill your tank with one to four big glasses of water (about 16 to 32 ounces) and do a minute's worth of resistance exercise. Choose from any of the following. Rotate your selections and aim to do a total of 3-5 one-minute daily sessions throughout the day.

Reverse Lunge: Stand with feet shoulder-width apart, arms at sides. Take one foot and step backward. Plant your toe firmly against the ground with the knee only slightly bent. Hold for a couple of seconds, maintaining your balance. Return to starting position and switch legs. Repeat for a minute.

Body Weight Squats: Stand with feet about shoulder-width apart, arms at sides or out in front of you. Bend knees, bringing your rear end down as if sitting on a chair. Raise and repeat. Do for a minute or as many as you can do consecutively, take a break and begin again until a count of 60 can be reached.

Standard Push-Up: Get down on the floor. Put your hands flat down, positioning them slightly wider than your shoulders, fingers pointed toward your head direction. Extend your arms and legs in a straight line. Feet can be close together or a bit wider depending upon what is most comfortable to you. Simultaneously raise yourself up onto your toes so you are balanced on your hands and toes. Keep your body in a straight line from head to toe, squeeze your butt and suck in your belly. This will help to prevent arching of your back. Inhale as you slowly bend your elbows and lower yourself until your elbows are at a 90-degree angle. Exhale as you push back up to the start position without locking your elbows, keeping them slightly bent. Repeat for as many repetitions as you can comfortably do in one minute, ideally building to 60-100 in a row. Start on your knees, doing all other parts the same if the regular full push-up is too hard at first.

Plank: See above and repeat all steps but simply hold the starting, top position. Do not dip down and up. Get into position and hold it for as long as you can, building up to a slow count of 60. You can also do this with your arm/elbow flat on the ground to start if you find the standard position too difficult.

Countertop Push-Up: Stand on toes two-three feet from the counter. Place hands on countertop, and lower down and get back up keeping elbows tight to your body. Start with 20 and aim to build up to a consecutive 60 repetitions. This is easier than a regular push-up and a good way to start for many. Once you've mastered these, move up to regular push-ups.

Standing Heel Raises: With feet together, rise up on your toes, then come down but only barely touching your heels to the ground. Tighten your buttocks as tightly as you can. Repeat for a count of 60 or as long as you can last.

Butt Squeezes: Lay down or stand and clench butt cheeks as tightly as possible. Relax and repeat 10-20 times. Do as often as possible.

Boxing Upper Cut: Get into a strong fighting position. Legs spread apart slightly wider than shoulder width with firmly bent knees. Tighten your abdominal muscles. Punch your right fist out to the left and then left fist out to the right. Alternate each arm for a count of 30. Then you can modify the movement slightly by imagining you are trying to knock the jaw of someone taller than you. Punch upward. Repeat for a count of 30 for each arm.

Basic Arm Spins: This one feels good and helps get muscles moving, making it a good warm-up. Stand with arms reaching out to the sides. Circle arms forward, keeping elbows straight and muscles in arms and belly tight and flexed. Aim for 30 repetitions circling forward and 30 repetitions circling backward.

Note: Even if you just alternate your 3-5 daily sessions between push-ups and body weight squats, you will be amazed by the results! Don't fret if you can only do your push-ups from the knee position—they will still be very effective for overall strengthening along with squats.

BASIC DUMBBELL ROUTINES

Lower Body: (By Far the MOST Important for Both Men & Women)

Squats: Squats can be done using just your own body weight or with dumbbells in each hand. Bend from knees until thighs are parallel to the ground (avoid letting knees turn inward). Keep back flat, lower back slightly arched in and head up, facing forward. Return to upright position and repeat 10 times.

Lunges: Holding the dumbbells at your sides, stand upright with feet shoulder-width apart. Step forward 2-4 feet with one foot and bend knee to about 90 degrees. Push off with front foot to return to starting position. Change legs and do 10 reps for each leg.

Calf Raises: Holding dumbbells at sides, stand upright with your feet shoulder-width apart. Go up and down on tippy toes rapidly for 10+ times. In a few days you may find you can do 60 or more in a minute.

Middle Body:

Supine Sit-Ups: Lay flat on a bed, couch, desk or floor and stretch arms straight back. Clasp hands and keeping legs and arms straight, bend up from the middle. Form a "U" but only go up as far as you can comfortably. Repeat 10 times. Add weight to hands when stronger.

Upper Body:

Simple Press: Stand and lift dumbbells over your head, keeping your body very straight. Lower the dumbbells slowly to shoulders. Push the dumbbells back up. Repeat 10 times.

Lateral Lift: Stand upright, knees bent, shoulder-width apart, hanging dumbbells together so they touch in front of you. Lift elbows like wings until elbows are 90 degrees and dumbbells are head-high. Slowly lower to start position and do 10 total. This exercise gives you those nicely cut "swimmers" shoulders.

Upright Rows or Underarm Lifts: Stand upright, feet shoulder-width apart, knees slightly bent. Keep dumbbells close to front or side of body and raise them to chin or under armpit. Slowly lower to start position and repeat 10 times.

Hammer Curls: Stand upright with dumbbells at sides. Bend elbows lifting dumbbells up and toward chest, turning palms inward so they face the body and touch the chest. Repeat 10 times.

Dumbbell Push-Ups: Place dumbbells on floor shoulder-width and parallel. Grip dumbbells with your hands and lower your chest and face to floor. Just before touching floor, push up and straighten arms. Repeat 10 times or see how many you can do.

Note: After 1-3 weeks, you will likely feel ready to raise your dumbbell weights. Men should switch to weights that allow only 6-8 repetitions at first, working up to 10. Women should switch to weights that allow 10-15 repetitions with effort required for the last three reps. After this, there is really no need to keep pushing for heavier weights. If it gets too easy and you really feel like it, go ahead and increase the weight or the repetitions.

A Mini-Bonus

The TurboCharged program has a lot of "mini". Perhaps we should have included Mini Coopers in our favorite car list! Along with mini-meals, mini-strength sessions and mini-challenges, another excellent mini-TurboCharging activity is jumping on a mini-trampoline (aka a "rebounder"). Rebounding is an excellent and easy activity that is proven to enhance immunity by stimulating your lymphatic system. Basically, your lymphatic system is a network of tubes—like the blood system, but without a pump. The system carries a fluid called lymph all around the body to help your cells cleanse themselves. The lymphatic system is part of the body's immune system and helps the body fight infection. Without getting carried away with a long explanation of why, what you need to know is that rebounding is one of the few activities that will "exercise" every cell in your body. The lymph cleansing that is triggered by rebounding is a good thing whether you're focused on losing excess fat or simply staying healthy and fit. Rebounding is also particularly beneficial to the veins in your legs, and regular use will improve and/or prevent varicose veins. We each use ours every morning for gentle, mini wake-up workouts of 5-10 minutes and often several more times during the day as time allows or if the weather is particularly bad outside. Five minutes is plenty and there is no need to break a sweat to reap the benefits. If you have one that has been collecting dust, polish it up and start bouncing. These are also a common yard sale item. So keep your eyes scouting for used ones, which are often resold for a fraction of their original cost.

Special Activity Note to Couch Potatoes or Those Tied to Their Desks...

If you have read this far, yet are still finding it impossible to imagine your life without a few hours of relaxing on the couch watching television or maybe claiming you simply can't get away from work...your excuses are still out! Every one of the exercises described above can be done while watching the tube, while on a conference call or along with whatever you do in your office. For example, you could do any of these without getting up from a chair:

- Suck your stomach in and hold tight for as long as you can. Release and breathe.

- Lift your legs straight out in front of you and hold steady for as long as you can. Release.

- Extend legs in front of you and criss-cross them like a scissors. Do as many as you can.

- Put your palms together in front of your chest and push tightly together as hard as you can. Hold for as long as you can push hard. Release and repeat.

- Extend your arms in front of you or to your sides at shoulder height. Pulse them up and down—up three inches, down three inches—as if you were flapping wings like a bird.

- Get off the couch during commercials and push-up, squat or lunge. The commercials are only trying to sell you truck-stop foods and junk that will take you off your road to success. Counter their messages with some healthful TurboCharging activity!

For every hour in front of a television, computer or desk, be sure to take one measly minute to tighten, flex and strengthen your muscles. Before you know it, you'll be able to do three minutes for every hour, and TV time will have become at least a little more productive. See www.turbo-charged.us.com for more exercises you can do in a chair.

TurboCharged on Schedule

You now have a series of steps to implement several times per day, whenever hunger arises and before you eat.

Ideally, you will benefit from establishing set times during the day; every two, three or four hours apart, so you begin the habit of "working the steps" before hunger has any chance to overwhelm your focus.

Time for a Review

- Drink 1-2 quarts of water within the first hour that you are up.

- Upon sensing any signs of hunger…

  ✔ Fill your tank with a large glass or two (think 16 to 32 ounces) of water again.

✔ Brush your teeth, rinse with mouthwash or suck on a breath-strip. Don't rinse.

✔ Get active doing anything. Get moving or take a walk. Even a brief 10 minutes of any activity is sufficient.

✔ Work your muscles. Do any one of the above TurboCharging routines for a minimum count of 20 or ideally doing as many as possible for one minute.

Following this sequence every 2-3 hours and before sleep tells the brain to:

- turn off your appetite;

- stay focused on using your body fat for energy;

- retain your muscle mass; and

- keep you TurboCharged.

In order for your brain to allow the burning of excess body fat for energy, it must first be assured that you need and want to maintain your muscles, your organs and your lean, vital tissues. Once this assurance is provided, the brain can be convinced that you no longer need or want to keep excess body fat. By day three of TurboCharging, if all steps are consistently followed as presented, and you eat the everyday foods you will learn about in Step #7, your brain will begin to cooperate as it turns to your body fat for energy while your muscles get finely toned and sleek. You will become TurboCharged.

Your body actually prefers to be in TurboCharged mode. The steps are designed so that your brain feels very satisfied. The wonderful effects can last a long time, sometimes four to five hours or more, which will naturally delay any sense of hunger since your body is happily feeding on your excess body fat. That said, we still recommend that you begin by establishing specific times in your day when you will work your steps. The reason we set two to three hour intervals for practicing these steps is that it is easier to prevent hunger pangs (as the steps do), than to test your willpower after they start voicing their cries.

TurboCharged...The "Write" Stuff

Helene Fisher recently turned 70 according to the calendar. Her Tanita body-fat scale now has her pegged at 56...and getting younger since she began TurboCharging a year ago.

Helene is a self-employed publicist and writer. She leads an extremely active, yet also stress-filled life that includes being caregiver to her chronically ill 80-year-old husband.

Helene had tried countless diets over the years, only to gain back the weight and experience subsequent disappointment. She always said, "I can do just fine all day...but I'm a nighttime eater. I just don't have the willpower come nightfall, and I don't know why."

Upon being introduced to the TurboCharged program, and learning about evening hunger and circadian rhythms, which we'll discuss in Step #7, she began first by simply committing to walk her two dogs a couple of times a day, drink lots of water and eat more fruit. These three steps alone triggered a quick five-pound weight loss, 1% decrease in body fat and a major gain in enthusiasm. Within two weeks, Helene was down a solid 11 pounds of body fat and she has not gained back an ounce, even though she admittedly gets caught up in the stress of the day and "hasn't really done too well incorporating the other steps."

Yet walking coupled with the TurboCharged foods has created a remarkable difference. Helene raves: "I've tried every diet program you can name. This time, even though I'm somewhat spotty with implementation, I haven't gained back any of the fat I've lost. I am amazed that I have hit a new low steady weight. More so, I know that as I stick with the steps, success is mine! I feel better than ever and my energy is boundless. I hope the world begins to TurboCharge!

Now, let us assure you, we realize that at some point you will have completed all the steps and be genuinely hungry. Let's look at what you might eat.

Step #7
Eating to TurboCharge

Right about now you might be wondering if you've read this far only to be told you need to brush your teeth, walk, keep active, drink water and live on your own body fat if you want to get sleek, lean and healthy. Let us assure you...TurboChargers eat. Real food, and plenty of it!

Please fasten your safety belt and pay attention. The race is about to start!

Start by Choosing Your Route

If you wanted to take a cross-country road-trip, there are a number of highways in addition to back roads that you could take to reach your destination. The route chosen would most likely be determined by how quickly you want to arrive, or whether you have the time and are inclined to take the more leisurely route to get to where you want to be.

Likewise, there are two ways to begin the TurboCharged program. You can get to your destination by following what we call the "Expressway," or you can get to the same destination but much faster by "putting the pedal to the metal," aiming to get to the finish line as quickly as possible, using the "SuperHighway" approach. Once you've arrived at the body-fat percentage that is ideal for your health, you will simply switch to "Cruise Control," which will be explained in a later chapter.

The road you take to the body you want is simply a personal preference. The difference, as you will learn, will get down to calories consumed within each 72-hour or three-day period. Taking the Expressway route, the calories are unlimited, assuming that you are selecting TurboCharged foods that we will outline. The SuperHighway introduces what we discussed back in Step #1, the concept of enlightened fasting, or eating highly nutritious foods but maximizing caloric consumption at 800 calories a day or less. Catch your breath and recover from your shock! We'll soon explain how this is actually very easy and even enjoyable.

An Important Request Before Continuing

Right now we have a simple request: Please take your time while you read this Step. It is long, introduces many new concepts, and might seem confusing at times. You need to read this entire section to fully understand why the TurboCharged way of living and eating will deliver rapid fat loss. If you skip around, you will miss something important that may make success elusive. It is also important to remind you that once you finish this and Step #8, the Question and Answer section should be read carefully, with your full attention, as it is designed to fill in the blanks and answer any questions that may be lingering. All the answers you need for a lifetime of leanness are between the covers of this book.

Finally, regardless of which road you choose, it is best if you do not just "drive right in" to TurboCharged eating without some preparation. Until you finish this book, we recommend that you continue to eat anything you want. When you are finished reading, you will be ready. For now, at the starting line, let's take a look at what you might eat to get you accelerating toward your personal goal.

A Few Significant Concepts

As we stated earlier, anyone, whether vegetarian, carnivore or cafeterian, can TurboCharge his or her body. However, when TurboChargers eat, they use a bit of evolutionary reasoning in their meal selections. Simply, it works like this: Our early ancestors, as we briefly discussed in Step #5, were on the run, fighting for survival. Most likely they were subsisting on very few calories consisting of easy to find and eat fruits, vegetables, seeds and maybe nuts along with other basic vegetation. Considering the energy requirements of their days, this was probably pretty close to what TurboChargers would call "enlightened fasting." Good nutrition, but not a heck of a lot of calories. At other times, when they were really lucky, early humans were chowing down, sometimes for days at a time, on whatever wild beast they managed to catch. Since there was no refrigeration, along with the fact that meats and organs of the wild beast kind were high in both proteins and fats, this food source would spoil rapidly. It is likely that animal food was eaten as a sole meal source until it was gone or too rotten to eat. Our early relatives didn't have the luxury of refrigeration, leisurely sitting down to eat and mixing a variety of foods as we do today. It simply wasn't practical or possible.

This bit of ancestral history gives us two good pieces of information.

First, it is highly likely that the body's digestive system did not evolve to eat many different foods at the same time—particularly protein/fat foods along with carbohydrates. The idea of eating balanced meals may look good on paper, but in the real world, these meals put too much stress on our digestive systems, plus they are the cause of indigestion and GERD or acid reflux. Our digestive system is really amazing and will attempt to deal with anything we put in our tanks, but this doesn't make balanced meals a good idea. Digesting food is hard work for our bodies, and ideally we want to keep digestion time to a minimum if we want maximum efficiency and performance. Your digestion and energy levels will improve enormously by practicing the TurboCharged guidelines you'll learn shortly. Without getting too scientific, suffice it to say that different food groups each require different digestive processes. Mixing carbohydrates with fats and/or proteins will result in the meal lingering in your stomach too long. This then creates indigestion and makes overall digestion of these meals more difficult, burdensome or even incomplete. Once you give TurboCharging a try for 10 days, you will be convinced that our recommendations are correct.

Second, an interesting question arises if one compares this kind of eating to dieters of today. Think about it. Our ancestors were either practically starving OR they were pigging out on massive amounts of fatty meat before it spoiled. You might think they'd be fat—like a yo-yo dieter who consumes low calories one day and then binges on large quantities of foods and calories the next when their willpower is shot. But history proves this isn't the case. Our ancestors didn't diet and they were not fat. Instead, they were active and lean. They ate by separating their nutrients (because they really had no choice.) To get and stay lean, TurboChargers do the same.

Choosing Your Meals

To accelerate the process of rapid fat burning, regardless of whether taking the Expressway, SuperHighway or Cruise Control route, TurboChargers eat one of six types of meals:

1) A meal with any amount of whole protein and/or fat alone or combined. This would include beef, fish, pork, venison, chicken, eggs, cheeses of all kinds and tofu.

2) A meal with any amount of fresh, whole fruits or vegetables. This includes baked potatoes, sweet potatoes, avocados and olives.

3) A meal of 90% whole protein and/or fat (as outlined in #1) along with no more than 10% vegetables. Think in terms of volume on a plate—not the calories of the food group.

4) A meal of 90% vegetables and/or fruits along with no more than 10% whole protein (as outlined in #1). Again, think in terms of volume on a plate—not calories of the food group. Use the "eye ball" rule.

5) A smoothie made with water (or ice) and a scoop of 100% whey, egg or pea protein powder that has no more than 3 grams of carbohydrate, about 25 grams of protein and approximately 100 calories per serving.*

6) A smoothie made with water (or ice) and 1-2 whole fruits and a scoop of 100% whey, egg or pea protein.*

*If you want to have a shake meal, the base liquid is always only water. If adding protein powder, the kind you choose is of utmost importance. First off, the protein powder must be protein "isolate" (i.e.: isolated or primarily protein) and should not have more than 3 grams of carbohydrate or 2 grams of fat per 20-25 grams of protein. Never use one with sugar or corn syrup. It is best to just use pure protein isolate, but it is OK if you find one that tastes good and is artificially flavored or sweetened.

TurboCharged meals are simple. Natural hygienists were the first to propose nutrient separation. They proposed that you should not eat a protein and a starchy carbohydrate in the same meal. This works wonders, particularly for indigestion. Irwin M. Stillman, MD, espoused eating either only protein meals for several weeks followed by vegetable based meals for weeks at a time. TurboChargers, however, take it to the next level. We ideally aim for entire meals of a single nutrient source exclusively. This triggers our bodies to burn the calories in the foods we eat much more efficiently, assures our brains that food is plentiful, facilitates digestion, and triggers the body to burn body fat for our excess energy requirements. This simple step helps move fat burning into warp speed.

Eating and Working with Body Rhythms

We all awaken dehydrated since our bodies continued working unbeknownst to us all night long. Knowing this, TurboChargers begin their day with 16 to 32 ounces of fresh water within the first hour of awakening. If they want a cup of coffee or tea, that's fine too after they fill their tanks with water. Once our bodies have cycled through natural easy awakening, which often includes the first bowel movement of the day, we go through our TurboCharged steps to confirm that it is true hunger we are experiencing. We get active, do a mini-muscle workout, or walk. Then we eat lightly—ideally fruits and/or vegetable meals—during daylight hours.

Due to evolutionary forces, our bodies react to circadian rhythms, which are natural wake-and-sleep patterns based on light. (Think: Early to bed, early to rise, makes a man *healthy*, wealthy and wise, or: The early bird catches the worm.) As a reaction to these natural light forces, most of us ebb toward sleepiness as the sun starts to set. This is also the very reason most dieters lose their willpower late in the day and why we may feel the strongest urge to snack, begin an evening meal that is more protein-centered and/or simply eat more food. Our body clock is sending sleep signals. Our busy lives are demanding that we stay up past our "natural" bedtimes. The end effect is that we all feel an equally natural strong urge to eat to keep our energy going into the evening.

As life is a constant series of cycles, TurboChargers work *with* the natural rhythms of a 24-hour day and use these patterns to rest, hydrate, eliminate, hydrate, move, nourish, hydrate, move, hydrate and nourish more intensely prior to the next rest. Did any other diet ever explain to you why you felt you had willpower during the day, but felt so hungry at night? Now you know it was circadian rhythm (your body's reaction to levels of light) that you were fighting, not a lack of willpower. Understanding these natural urges to eat more in the late afternoon and evening, TurboChargers find balance and peace as they have learned to stop resisting natural rhythms and patterns and instead work with them. So again, working with these patterns, TurboChargers save their heavier, protein meals for the evenings.

When initiating the TurboCharged program, if you find you are still hungry after a meal, even if it was a high-protein meal and you topped off your tank sufficiently with plenty of water, TurboChargers eat a dessert of whole fruits until satiated. You could certainly have unlimited vegetables too, but they likely won't satisfy a "sweet-tooth" memory although they will trigger satiety hormones. If you can delay this "dessert," using it as a meal an hour or two later, this would be better, but if not, that's okay.

You can eat more TurboCharged foods than you are normally used to—especially fruit. Use fruit anytime to cut off appetite. Don't limit yourself, think quantity: as many as three to five apples, bananas, pears, peaches, melons or any other fruits you like would be just fine. If you get an urge, try to fill up on fruit, ideally eating it alone as a sole food source of a meal. Buy a bunch of fruit and get it all washed, chilled and ready to eat. Always have plenty on hand. Don't stop eating until you feel full. Remember, as we said earlier, it is virtually impossible to overeat on fruit. Watermelon, so often incorrectly cited as a high-sugar, anti-diet food, is actually a great example of both a high-water food that naturally effects stomach expansion and triggers the release of satiety hormones. World-renowned Paleolithic expert Loren Cordain, Ph.D. and his team determined in a study that most people would stop eating watermelon after about three pounds, which would equal about 435 calories of food, or even 6 pounds (870 calories) because their stomach volumes simply cannot take more food. This example pretty much sums up why TurboChargers rely on fruit for feeling satisfied and full after doing all the steps, when we are hungry.

Days filled with fruits and/or vegetables will help increase the hormone glucagon in your body to ensure a steady supply of energy. When glucagon is present, most of your body's energy is derived from a mix of glycogen reserves and fat stores. At the same time, the lower insulin levels that ensue, allow growth hormone (GW) to peak. When your levels of growth hormone increase, your body's capacity to burn fat, as well as rejuvenate and repair tissues, also increases. Although we will all grow old and die, we firmly believe that this program, by "manipulating" your hunger and getting it to work for your health and longevity instead of against you, significantly slows the process of aging.

Fruits will make transitioning your body into TurboCharged status much easier, and you may find that you immediately look and feel better simply by adding more fresh fruit to your daily diet.

For anyone who has struggled with dieting in the past, eating fruit is critical. Our taste buds are damaged from incorrect diets and not eating enough TurboCharged foods, particularly fruits, so when starting a diet you may crave junk foods. Consider this the best reason to stuff yourself with fruit! Plus, you'll be eating nutrition-packed, water-filled foods that are very healthful. In their whole natural state, fruits are deliciously sweet and satisfying.

As you work the TurboCharged program, you will notice you desire less and less food. Your engine is beginning to function properly again as it uses your body fat for fuel. By all means please COOPERATE! Go with the feeling. Enjoy eating when you are truly hungry and eat till you are satisfied. Keep yourself busy. Rinse your mouth and brush your teeth. Stay active. Before you know it—you will be TurboCharged and driving quickly toward your personal finish line in a healthier and leaner body.

Before we talk about how TurboChargers can really rev up and race to reach their goal of a sleek physique more quickly than any other diet before…

Have You Noticed What TurboChargers Do <u>Not</u> Eat?

TIME FOR A PIT STOP…

TurboChargers do not eat refined foods in any form and they drive right by any and all grain products. Let's look at why.

The Pancreas, Insulin and Food Connection

Your body was not designed to handle excess and/or concentrated carbohydrates. When overconsumed, refined carbohydrates flood the body with too much glucose (sugar). To deal with the excess glucose, your pancreas secretes the hormone insulin. Most of this excess glucose is converted to body fat. Your pancreas becomes overworked by trying to deal with this constant supply of sugar. During the past 60 years an emphasis has been placed on low-fat foods. As a result the intake of sugars, grains and grain-based products has gone up dramatically (all of which overwork and stress your pancreas and other bodily functions). Cancer, diabetes, heart disease, allergies and immunity-related conditions have skyrocketed. In every civilization from Egypt until today, when grains and other refined foods are (were) eaten in great quantity and/or in combination with other foods, obesity and disease become more common. Even Asian countries are now hitting record levels of obesity and disease. Now that sugar is in virtually every food and grains are so "in-grained" in the modern diet, the result is a massive assault on our delicate physiology, which was not designed to consume so many insulin-triggering foods.

The Complexity of Complex Carbohydrates

There is a tendency in all dietary literature to lump together fruits, vegetables, beans, nuts, legumes, cereals and grains in the catchall food category of "complex carbohydrates." This is very convenient for makers of any kind of bread, cereal and cereal bars and very bad for consumers, especially TurboChargers.

Refined sugar consumption has risen exponentially in the West and there appears to be no sign of a ceiling. Today we consume more refined carbohydrates and sugar than ever. Sugar alone is now consumed at over twice the rate of 75 years ago. Fat-free products line grocery store shelves. Sugar is now not just sugar. It has fancy names like high-fructose corn syrup that is effectively identical to sugar in its chemical makeup despite being marketed heavily as a "healthy" sugar. It's not! This is false. Then add in things like malt, corn syrup and good old-fashioned molasses. "Health" food stores and manufacturers claim that agave nectar, brown rice syrup, barley malt, brown sugar and organic evaporated cane juice are healthier sugars too. They are not! Sugar by any other name is still sugar. This includes malt dextrin, dextrose, xylitol, maltose, starch and syrups, to name a few. Regardless of the name a manufacturer might choose in order to confuse you, any and all sugar causes the same kinds of detrimental effects to your body.

Adults in the US are now estimated to be consuming about 130 pounds of refined sugars annually. Let's share a visual on this: The next time you go to a grocery store, pick up a one- pound box of sugar. The average American consumes the equivalent of two or more of these boxes every week. Quite staggering, isn't it!

More frightening is the fact that these figures reach a whopping average of 274 pounds annually for our children! That is about five pounds a week! Surely you'd never let a child eat that in a bag of sugar. We are inadvertently setting the stage for our children to become obese adults. "How does this happen?" you might ask.

Most of us want to be healthy and we certainly don't want to inflict harm on our children. We may even try hard to avoid obvious sugar foods. Well, there's the problem. Sugar today is not as obvious on the ingredient list as it once was. Sugar is hidden in our food. You just don't see it. Seventy-five percent of the sugar we consume is in the processed foods we buy at stores or in restaurants, and only 25% percent is added directly at home.

We all know, even if we sometimes don't want to admit it, that sugar is plentiful in cookies, cakes, pie, doughnuts, ice cream, powdered or pre-made flavored water drinks, candy bars, soft drinks, gelatin, jam, syrup, salad dressings, pudding and most other prepared foods. But did you know this? Sugar is even in most commercial French fries. It is also hidden under any number of names in most cereals, yogurts, ketchups, salad dressings, soups and even vitamins and medications.

Sugar is creeping into our bodies, insidiously destroying our health and making us fatter and fatter. Consequently, we are turning ourselves and our children into diabetics in mind-boggling numbers. Along with all this sugar is our massive grain consumption of wheat, rice and oats, for example, as well as the countless "foods" that grains are processed into: breads, cereals, snack/health bars, etc. Grains are also a major contributor to the problems of obesity and ill health.

Grains Are Poor Body Fuels

Contrary to what you may have heard about eating grains for energy, all grains are imperfect fuel for your body's energy requirements. All grains, whole or otherwise, are processed and are very low in natural water content while also being low in essential vitamins, minerals, phytochemicals and micronutrients. Whole grains also contain a substance called phytate that almost entirely prevents the absorption of any calcium, iron or zinc that is found in whole grains. Any processing of a grain only pushes them down the healthful food chain, depleting the limited natural water of the grain while destroying most if not all nutrients. By now you probably realize that water and the water content in food are vital aspects of TurboCharging. A steak actually has higher water content than brown rice. Surprised? Grains and grain-based products are not TurboCharging foods! To make matters worse, we are snacking on these sugary, fat-sugar grain-based combos more than ever. *The American Journal of Clinical Nutrition* recently reported that we are consuming more snacks than meals. The average adult consumed roughly 200 calories from snacks in the mid-1970s, 360 calories in the mid-1990s, and 470 in the latest survey. The average child consumed roughly 240 calories from snacks in the mid-1970s, 420 calories in the mid-1990s, and 500 calories of junk each day in the latest survey! Plus, sugar-laden beverages are quenching the thirst caused by these dehydrating foods and are now contributing an average of 420 calories per day in the average adult's diet, up from 290 calories in the 1970s. These calories for children are undoubtedly even higher.

This chart appeared in the March 2009 edition of *Reader's Digest*. Note: Not a single grain or processed grain food was listed as a vital nutrient provider.

EAT YOUR VITAMINS*:

Vitamin C	Vitamin E	Beta-carotene	Folate	B6	B12
• Broccoli	• Almonds	• Carrots	• Lentils	• Bananas	• Clams
• Red Bell Pepper	• Sunflower Seeds	• Pumpkin	• Garbanzo Beans	• Garbanzo Beans	• Rainbow Trout
• Brussels Sprouts	• Hazelnuts	• Spinach	• Asparagus	• Chicken	• Sockeye Salmon
• Papaya	• Sunflower Oil	• Sweet Potato	• Black beans		• Beef
	• Peanut Butter		• Oranges		

* No grains required!

More Bad News for Sugar and Grains...

Remember, if you are not TurboCharged, your body is constantly running on sugar supplied by the food you eat and drink.

Your pancreas releases insulin in an effort to control the levels of sugar in your blood. TurboChargers understand that the constant consumption of highly processed and refined foods (sugar, grains and their derivative products) causes insulin-related pathologies because the pancreas was never designed to deal with these kinds of food, cannot sustain high insulin production and tissues cannot adequately respond long term to consistently high insulin levels. Hypertension, diabetes, dyslipidemia, cardiovascular disease, obesity, and high and low blood sugar all result when the body has to battle against chronically high insulin levels. Insulin-related pathologies alter cellular proliferation and are now the likely cause of pre-teen girls developing breasts and getting their periods before age 13, as well as some types of cancer, polycystic ovary syndrome, myopia, acne and even male vertex balding. We are now raising an entire generation on the "benefits" of the USDA Food Pyramid. Children are being taught that the bulk of their dietary calories should consist of grains and breads first and foremost for energy. This is horrifying on at least two levels: First, consider the fact that obesity, diabetes and heart disease are all up since the introduction of this theory in the early 1960s. At that time we ate more meat and fat, yet obesity affected less than 1% of the US population. Clearly with over 30% of our population at obese levels, something is grossly wrong. Second, prescriptions for hyperactivity and attention deficit for both children and adults are at mind-boggling highs. Why isn't anyone asking if we, and especially our children, really need all the added sugar and grains for extra energy?

Statistics prove we are fighting a major battle if we want to regain our TurboCharged status. Government-sponsored studies and other marketing results show that the dominant foods of the decade will be snack foods, frozen foods, plastic-wrapped pre-prepared full meal foods and microwaveable foods. Bakery sections in grocery stores are expanding. Many meat and fish products or dishes are being offered as "pre-prepared" instead of simply and naturally. This increases our risk of ingesting all kinds of additives that will not contribute to our health, leading with sugar to sweeten things up, salt, gravy and other fatty-sauce accompaniments. Heavily pro-cessed "heat and eat" foods are increasingly being marketed. A walk through any grocery store readily confirms this.

Carbohydrates and carbohydrate/fat combinations of foods that do not have a naturally high water content, basically anything other than fruits and vegetables, will trigger an over-release of insulin to combat the resulting spike in our blood sugar. Our bodies must compensate. We store the excess sugar by putting a little in our muscles and liver as glycogen. The rest gets warehoused as visible body fat, as well as dangerous internal fat that develops around our vital organs. Every grain product counts as a refined carbohydrate, even those touted as "whole" grain. Any and all refined carbohydrates in our diets will keep this vicious cycle going, and fat will continue to accumulate. The only exception might be folks in that elite group who manage to do 60-90 minutes of aerobics daily, and even they are racing uphill, against the wind and with an empty tank!

Following "expert" advice and regularly eating grain-based products spread out over the course of your day, even in small amounts, will shut down your TurboCharger and make fat loss almost impossible.

Are you sure grains aren't good for me?

Here is a summary of the salient facts regarding grains.

1) Grains are a relatively recent addition to the human diet, when compared to our species' lifespan, and are not necessary if adequate amounts of fresh foods are available.

2) Commercial breads eaten today contain virtually no nutritive properties, cannot support animal life and are full of chemicals. (See the full history of grains at www.turbocharged.us.com)

3) Breakfast cereals have had any original nutrients mashed, processed and squashed out of them only to be put back in as "fortified" synthetic vitamins… and are generally composed of 25-50% or more sugar.

4) "Fortified" grain products are useless, deceptive and serve no real nutritional need.

5) When refined grains are eaten, vitamins and minerals already present in your body are depleted.

6) Modern breads that include dozens of additives, preservatives and fragmented food forms, cause multi-toxic conditions while setting the stage for obesity and disease.

7) It is very dehydrating to your body to process grains.

8) Grains are the most calorically dense foods, ounce per ounce.

People do not understand the extent to which grains impact our health and weight. We are fed studies that show better health from eating whole grains, but unfortunately it is because these diets are compared only to regular Western diets and not to the diets of populations that consume no grains at all. The latter are far healthier than those so-called healthy grain-eating groups in their studies. Eat grains at your own health peril. They are never going to support a TurboCharged sleek and lean physique or the long-term functioning of your health.

The take-away facts regarding grains and sugar are simple:

- Your body processes all grain products, refined carbohydrates and fat/sugar combo foods as sugar.

- These products trigger high insulin release.

- This results in the continual storage of excess sugar as body fat.

- Remove all sugar and grain-based carbohydrates to begin the conversion of stored body fat into energy for activity and all other bodily processes.

- The result: TurboCharging begins and you move rapidly down the road to a fabulous and healthy body!

NOW, LET'S PULL OUT OF THIS PIT STOP AND GET BACK ON THE ROAD...

TurboCharging to Win the Race

A TurboCharged diet, along with all the steps we have presented, will result in a body-fat loss of 2% or more per week. This will equate to 2-7 pounds of body fat or "weight" depending on how consistent you are and how much extra fat you started with. You never have to count calories and you can eat as much as you want.

Let's review: TurboChargers choose either a protein meal or a carbohydrate meal (fruits and/or vegetables) without mixing them. If any mixing is done, TurboChargers eat 90% protein (including meat, chicken, tofu, cheese, eggs or fish) and 10% carbohydrate, made up of only fruits and/or vegetables. (Once you have reached your Cruise Control weight, proteins can also include beans and nuts.) OR: You can have a meal consisting of 90% fruits and/or vegetables with only about 10% protein. However, 100% of either food group is best: all protein or all fruits and/or vegetables in any meal. When using the 90%-10% option, just eyeball the portions by approximating the volume of the food, using your best judgment. Make sure to eat at least one all protein meal within any three-day period and use whole proteins. Protein has two to three times the thermal effect of either fats or carbohydrates, which simply means this: Eating protein as directed in *TurboCharged* will rev up your metabolism and speed your fat loss.

Regardless of the meal you choose, begin and follow any meal with 16 to 32 ounces of non-caloric fluid. No extra fluid is necessary after 6 pm.

It is important to note and quite contrary to most other diet recommendations—particularly low-carbohydrate programs—that there is no amount of fruit that would be considered too much if you are eating whole, fresh fruit as your food choice every single day. Overeating on fresh fruits alone is pretty hard to do. The exception would be dried fruits, which lack sufficient water and are therefore highly concentrated doses of sugar. Additionally, it is important to remember that fruit is a food that is best consumed alone. On an empty stomach and as the sole type of food ingested, the nutrients and water naturally occurring in fruit will be assimilated into the body both rapidly and efficiently. However, when fruit is combined with other high-fat foods such as nuts, seeds, cheese or fatty meats in high quantity, fat will begin to accumulate.

After reading this book, if you ate ONLY fruit after 7 pm and did just this one thing, you would dramatically improve your health and energy.

Dian TurboCharges her body by starting each day with a few big glasses of water around 6 am. She tries to catch the sunrise, while bouncing on her rebounder for five to ten minutes before the rest of her house awakens. After getting her kids off to school, she takes a brisk 30 to 45 minute walk of 6,000 or more steps prior to work whenever possible. The day continues with drinking lots of water, sipping a small cappuccino with half-and-half or plain hot tea in the morning, a round of mini-muscle workouts or rebounding mid-morning. Starting at about 11 am-noon she begins eating fruit until satisfied or a vegetable salad if she is out at a business lunch. The afternoon is filled with fruit or veggies, plenty of water, one minute of squats and a minute of push-ups every two hours throughout the afternoon and evening, random activities and minty mouth-washing. (She is known to participate on conference calls while bouncing on her rebounder.) Late afternoon or early evening she likes to eat a good homemade guacamole made with a couple of avocados and salsa that is scooped up with endive "chips", or nuts, or a frittata or omelet made with a couple of eggs and fresh herbs or maybe a piece of fish with some veggies or a hearty salad and steamed vegetables if in a restaurant. So FYI: Don't listen to anyone who tells you to avoid avocados or nuts because of their high calorie and fat content! They are excellent Cruise Control maintenance foods. Dian is evidence that such foods in their raw state might actually accelerate fat burning, and according to her body-fat scale, reduce biological aging. The remainder of her night winds down with assisting in homework, catching up with her husband and reading her favorite kinds of books along with a soothing drink consisting of a cinnamon stick in hot water (good heart antioxidants) or a mint tea. If she gets the urge for more food or something sweet and tasty, she fills up on all kinds of ripe, fresh fruit. She doesn't count calories, or carbohydrates or grams of protein or fat. She stays lean and TurboCharged by following all the steps, including 3-5 mini-muscle routines throughout the day, lots of activity plus walking and eating TurboCharged foods whenever she is hungry.

Tom takes an entirely different approach. Whenever he is in the mood to get very cut and lean, he quickly incorporates the following routine. First thing upon awakening he jumps on his rebounder for five minutes immediately followed by a set of push-ups. After that, he drinks one quart of water and two cups of black coffee. He sets his internal alarm clock for every two hours and will do a set of body-weight squats, pull-ups or push-ups (rotating between the three). When true hunger arises, he makes a smoothie consisting of a scoop of whey protein in water or eats a piece of fruit, depending on which satisfies his urge. This schedule continues all day. Dinner is either a large salad with fresh lemon (and perhaps a teaspoon of really good olive oil) or a piece of broiled or poached fish or a can of sardines. (He loves sardines.) If he is hungry later in the evening (after doing another mini-set) he will have another scoop of protein powder or a frozen banana. He also walks as much as his schedule allows. His cruise control days are very similar activity-wise, but food-wise, he skips the protein powder and instead opts to eat plenty of the whole foods included in the TurboCharged meal guidelines, namely meats, fish, chicken, cheeses and lots of vegetables and fruits.

Ignore the Calories

When you begin, calories should be ignored. At the start-ing line, the most important things are food separation and unlimited amounts of fruits, followed by vegetables and a protein meal daily or at a minimum once every three days. Once you begin to TurboCharge your body and regain performance after the first few days or so, you will notice hunger disappearing.

You will naturally start consuming what is known as a very low-calorie diet (VLCD) as you become quite comfortable with the lack of hunger that will ensue once your brain adjusts to the idea of sourcing your excess body fat for its energy needs rather than constant sugar from your current diet. Increasingly lengthy periods without food will naturally pass because your brain will have become content sourcing body fat as long as you are preserving lean body mass with the other TurboCharged steps.

A Loss of Appetite…

Initially, you may find you have very high food volume days using the TurboCharged foods, but you will soon find that you naturally tend to go days at a time consuming a very meager supply of food. You don't have to cut food quantities—it just seems to happen. Some TurboChargers report that they do not feel like eating at all. As we discussed earlier, we don't recommend traditional fasting. The TurboCharged foods supply excellent nutrition for your body and are important to your ultimate high-performance and health objectives, even if your meals on some days are just a few fruits and/or a can of tuna for the day with lots of water, accompanied by all the other steps.

It is our experience that to most TurboChargers, it becomes very natural to know whether or not they need a whole protein meal or a fruit/vegetable meal. Within about 10 days of following the program strictly and not haphazardly, you will notice a personal rhythm starting to develop. "Crash meals," those that trigger high insulin production, will really slow down your progress and performance during the first few 10-day cycles and may prevent you from reaching a TurboCharged state altogether.

Of course everyone has "off" meals, including us. Sometimes it takes a really off meal to motivate oneself even more. That has been true with virtually all TurboChargers and us.

Start out by committing to be disciplined and focused for 10 days. If you do the TurboCharged program as outlined in these pages, we can assure you that it becomes virtually impossible to not become very motivated by the results. Regardless of the amount of body fat you need to lose, 10 days will make a huge difference in how you feel and look!

After completing each 10-day cycle, some TurboChargers plan an off day. However, we have found it quite interesting, and observed this ourselves, that all report that their favorite past indulgences seem to have lost some of their thrill, and worse, many notice bloating and gas, general discomfort and sometimes even a bit of undesirable edginess. Consequently, their next cycle gets even better, as they typically realize they like how they are feeling and also no longer want to slow their fat-burning momentum.

TurboChargers Know...Excuses are O U T!

"I've been so busy and had work stress and had to go to a business dinner and had to have the tasty cookies and candies over the holidays and had children and family pulling me in six different directions and had a big project to complete and had a big problem come up..." And on and on it goes.

Excuses are officially out! It is too easy to incorporate TurboCharged into your lifestyle. You have a goal. Get to sleek, lean and healthy first. Cross your personal "finish line." Make sure your body fat is within the recommended ranges. Remember, you have dangerous visceral fat that you can't see inside your body, around vital organs.

Win your personal championship race first and make history for yourself and all who follow you. You will become a winner in our culture. Unique, stronger minded, better able to accomplish any goal. Best of all...you will look and feel like a younger woman or man.

Hidden Roadblocks to Success

Now you know that the best TurboCharged meals are either 100% protein (meat, fish, eggs, cheese or tofu) OR 100% fruits or vegetables OR a combination of fruits and vegetables OR a 90/10 combo. You will slow down and risk dropping from the race if you start combining different foods. Worse, you may crash if you add grains, gravies, dressings and such to your meals. Fat mixed with carbohydrate is particularly problematic and most likely will result in accruing those calories as body fat. Keep meals simple. Don't forget this rule.

Have your fruits without fat and vegetables in any quantity with limited fat. If you feel the need for some fat with your veggies, slice up a succulent, tasty avocado alone or toss it in a blender with some tomatoes and onions to create your own healthful dressing. Enjoy your eggs, cheese, beef or fish while including very few or no vegetables or fruits during the meal. Protein combined with fat is a natural combination, so whole proteins are great at any meal. However, if you add carbohydrate to that meal other than a small quantity of vegetables or fruits, that meal will likely end up increasing your body fat.

It is OK to do a small amount of combining protein and carbohydrates — if you do one or the other sparingly and stick with fruits and veggies as the sole form of carbohydrate. When you do so, stick with the recommended 90/10% eyeball rule.

Yogurt and Milk

As you have already seen, TurboChargers may eat cheese, which counts as a protein/fat source. For some, adding a little cheese once in awhile seems to provide just enough tasty fat and variety to keep on track. Milk, yogurt and most other dairy products, however, are too high in lactose (sugar) and they tend to stimulate the hyper-production of insulin, which is the very thing we are trying to reduce. There may be some nutritional value in yogurt, but for losing body fat there is too much combining of fat (milk fat) and sugar (lactose) in most dairy products. And as you now know—fat/

sugar or fat/carbohydrate are the absolute WORST culprits for adding body fat.   Most yogurt has lactose plus lots of extra sugar added (usually one of the top three ingredients listed on the label).   Since so many parents consider yogurt a great breakfast food, despite its extraordinarily high sugar content, this may explain why so many kids are having problems paying attention at school.   The sugar load is simply too much and the fat/sugar combo is predisposing our children to obesity. If the yogurt is the "Greek" style product, high in protein and fat and very low in lactose, it could be considered a viable protein/fat—assuming it is plain with no sugar added. However, TurboChargers who love eating yogurt should save it for Cruise Control mode and always be careful to read the label, watching for any added sugar.

Although milk contains calcium and other nutrients, it, too, will delay your progress. Skim milk is way too high in sugar, and whole milk mixes fat and carbohydrate. We generally do not lose minerals like calcium unless we are eating too many breads, pastas, grains or other acid-forming foods (primarily junk foods) and not enough alkalinizing foods (think fruits and vegetables) and/or we are not stressing our muscles and bones with some form of resistance activity. The mini-weight work and foods you are eating on the TurboCharged program will provide everything you need to prevent mineral and bone loss. This plan works much better than any supplements or drugs. If you want something in your coffee or tea, limit your liquid dairy to no more than two tablespoons of half-and-half, ideally recording it as a mini-fat meal. Don't combine this kind of coffee drink with fruit—or you will be inadvertently ingesting a fat/carbohydrate combo and temporarily flipping off your fat-burning switch.

Both of these regularly recommended "diet" foods drive insulin levels higher. High insulin levels increase the odds of crashing and burning the absolute best intentions.

Vital Food Groups—Getting Them All in a Sample Day...

- Water—lots of it. Start the day with a few big glasses. Then fill your tank every 2-3 hours.

- Leafy greens and yellow, orange, green and red vegetables. Color delivers both nutrients and faster TurboCharging performance. Always think color when preparing salads.

- Fruits and Berries. Nature's perfect dessert and sweet-tooth satiator.

- Lean Meats, Poultry, Eggs, Seafood, Beans, Tofu. Vital protein for moods, tissue repair and maintenance and strength.

- Cheese and Olive Oil—because a little bit of fat is tasty and helps TurboChargers stay on track.

    NOTE: Nuts are super-nutritious, but during the SuperHighway phase of TurboCharged, they may slow or halt your progress altogether unless your diet is high in vegetables and lower in fruits. The natural carbohydrates (sugars) in fruits, coupled with the natural fats in nuts, combine to turn off the fat-burning switch and keep the body running on sugar. While trying to reduce body fat, sprinkle raw nuts or seeds very sparingly on a salad or have a small handful with protein meals. Once you have reached your body fat percentage goal, feel free to indulge in the raw, unsalted nuts of your choice. Nuts are wonderful, tasty, fiber-filled foods. Now that we are TurboCharged we eat them by the pound, as a sole source food meal, with no detrimental effects.

Racing to the Finish Line via the TurboCharged SuperHighway

At this point, you know that much of our well-researched health philosophy runs counter to common advice. We will mention one more bit of it here: "You must lose weight slowly or you will gain it back."

To this, we have a simple response: Wrong! Speed up and drive quickly to your personal fat-loss finish line. Do not pull over and do not stop! You will be inspired, proud and envied by all. Others will stop and stare as you cruise by in your new sleek and fabulous physique. Why would you want to delay that reward even a single split second?

On the flipside, for opponents of extremely rapid fat loss, we submit this argument: If someone could improve their health sooner rather than later, or if one is seriously obese, diabetic, facing surgery or dealing with any other comparable life-threatening scenario, what is really more drastic? Losing body fat rapidly with strong conviction and willpower, or psychologically setting oneself up for failure—knowing it could take many months or years to lose the unhealthy body fat and possibly committing to open heart surgery, a potential amputation of a limb from diabetic ulcers, or a lifetime of illness, pain and medications? We submit that rapid loss of excess, hurtful body fat, done the TurboCharged way, is the healthiest route for virtually everyone.

The SuperHighway approach to TurboCharged is differentiated from the Expressway by days where only 300-800 total calories are consumed over a 24-hour period. This is what we call "enlightened fasting." These calories consist of eating the real foods we discussed earlier, in any of the six combinations outlined. The more calories you consume the longer it takes to reach your finish line. Eight hundred calories per day seems to be the very high-end number for speedy results. Note: Any time you exceed your actual daily calorie requirements, regardless of what you are eating, you will gain weight. Your body-fat scale will help guide you with this. If you are not seeing results or they are not coming as quickly as you would like, eat less!

We know this sounds hard to believe: Only 300-800 calories for a whole day! Are we crazy? This is simply a road you choose to travel if you want to really experience the trip.

Calorie restriction has beneficial effects and this has been known for a very long time. How do we know this? Over 2,000 animal studies since the 1930s, and hundreds of human studies, show that extreme calorie restriction improves health and increases longevity. For over 80 years, scientific research has demonstrated that periods of starvation return insulin sensitivity in Type 2 diabetics and result in resistance to many diseases. The highly respected Mayo Clinic has published numerous studies supporting the benefits of controlled starvation. Very low-calorie diets (VLCD) are the most studied diets in the world. There are more than 2,000 scientific papers supporting the beneficial aspects of severe calorie restriction, not only for weight loss, but also for overall long-term health. Counter-claims to VLCDs are simply unsubstantiated. Do you know the best part of a nutritionally replete VLCD or "enlightened fasting" as we call it? When calories are held to the lower ranges, and the nutrition quotient of foods eaten is held in the optimally high ranges, there is little to no hunger, more energy, greater willpower and far more rapid fat loss. Your body becomes much more efficient at using its excess fat for energy and does this even more so when all the Steps are followed as outlined within these pages.

The basic problem today is that people simply eat too much and also make bad food choices. Individually, each presents its own problems. Moving to correct food choices and avoiding sugars and processed foods while restricting or eliminating grains will have considerable beneficial effects alone.

By making correct food choices and eating minimal calories while following the SuperHighway approach along with all the TurboCharged steps, fat loss is maximized while your body's efficiency is greatly increased. As a result, you are not hungry and feel wonderful. When you are making correct food choices and eating the proper quantity, there is no need for supplements. Just follow the program as outlined and the results will be obvious and speak for themselves.

We know it may be hard to believe that this is possible. We too dealt with initial shock at the thought of consuming less than 800 calories daily, which was then followed by sheer joy at the results. There is virtually no hunger when the TurboCharged steps are implemented three to five times a day along with consuming TurboCharged meals as outlined.

To drop excess fat in record time, TurboChargers taking the SuperHighway find it is best to:

- Be very strict and eat at least 300 calories to a maximum of 800 calories per day, selecting only from TurboCharged foods for 4-5 days.

- Throw in a higher-calorie (free) day every 4-5 days while continuing to eat only TurboCharged foods— just simply eat more of them.

- Follow every other Step in intervals a maximum of 2-3 hours apart.

This pattern breaks things up while providing flexibility for various dining commitments (if you plan ahead). Intermittent large meals actually help to keep your metabolism revved up. The best way to lose body fat while increasing metabolism is by being "random". Just don't do consecutive high-calorie (free) days or even consecutive high-calorie meals if you want to lose body fat rapidly.

**Flexibility of Menu Selection Is Yours... An Incomplete Sample Selection
SuperHighway, Expressway and Cruise Control Foods**

Meat (lean)	Avocados	Olives
Most Wild Game	Broccoli	Cauliflower
Poultry	String Beans	Turnips
Seafood	Asparagus	Cucumber
Fish	Radishes	Spinach
Eggs	Summer Squash	Cabbage
Cheese	Mushrooms	Onions
Olive Oil	Celery	
Sour Cream & Chives	Lemon/Juice	Apples
Tofu	Lettuces of All Kinds	Melons
Water	Brussels Sprouts	Berries
	Tomatoes	Plums

Expressway and Cruise Control Foods include all of the above, plus:

Carrots
Coconut
Peas
Rutabagas
Winter Squash
Pumpkin
Cherries
Peaches

Cruise Control Foods:
**Include all of the above, plus these nutritiously perfect foods that
will keep energy soaring for athletes and children, while helping to
maintain your TurboCharged physique once you reach your goal.**

Apricots
Dates
Bananas
Beans
Beets
Corn (fresh or whole...not chips!)
Parsnips
Yams
Potatoes (see corn)
Nuts and Natural Nut Butter

Base Metabolic Rate and TurboCharging

At this point, after introducing the SuperHighway, "enlightened fasting" approach to rapid body-fat loss, we are often asked, "Won't eating a mere 800 calories or less a day lower my Base Metabolic Rate (BMR)?

We can firmly say with conviction: Absolutely NOT! Unless you fail to follow all of the Steps as directed. In fact, once you are TurboCharged you may find yourself consuming more calories than ever before, yet continually noticing that your body is reshaping itself, continuing to make you look more defined, lean and sleek. The reason this happens is that TurboCharged includes the steps for muscle retention along with encouraging maximum hydration to trigger fat burning for energy. Working your muscles, along with taking in adequate hydration as presented in this program, kickstarts your metabolism into hyperdrive and keeps it there.

Base Metabolic Rate (BMR) is best understood as the energy needed to keep normal body processes going. Your BMR depends on factors like height, weight, amount of muscle and bone, age and sex. It is identified as the number of calories required on a daily basis to keep your lean body mass constant. Fewer calories will likely result in weight (not necessary fat) loss and more calories will lead to weight (or fat) gain depending on the source of those calories. The body requires energy at all times, including when sleeping, keeping the heart beating, lungs breathing, kidneys working, cells repairing, new tissues building, and heat generating to keep body temperature steady, as well as to support the vast networks that circulate messages and pump nutrient-rich blood and remove waste. *Loss of lean muscle mass results in a lower BMR.* In other words, the amount of calories you need to maintain your weight will keep going down if you keep depleting your muscle mass.

Highly stressful lifestyles and exhausting regimens of aerobics and/or weight training can deplete your lean muscle mass, further lowering BMR. High protein, low-fat and low-calorie diets will all result in loss of lean muscle tissue. TurboCharged is different in that we use the separation of whole proteins and fat from fruits and vegetables while avoiding grains and refined foods whenever possible to accomplish fat loss and promote health. Further, we recommend walking, along with mini-weight workouts 3-5 times daily, to keep your indispensable muscle tissue vital and strong. This holistic combination keeps your BMR revving high.

Satisfying TurboCharged Meals

A nutritionally replete meal of 100 calories, like some fruit, vegetables, a piece of meat or a chunk of cheese, for example, is just enough to send a message to your brain that food is available—assuming this is coupled with a few big glasses of water, a walk and/or a mini-weight-bearing activity. As we said earlier, this program must be worked in its entirety for results. Why? Each step works together to remind your brain that you are alive, well, need your muscles and have plenty of body fat for fuel.

When you begin TurboCharging it is helpful to eat something (50-200 calories) every couple of hours whenever you feel hungry. Drinking a sufficient quantity of water regardless of whether you eat or not is important because it fills the stomach. When trying to get to the finish line in record time, TurboCharged portions should be about 100 calories per serving but can still range from 50-200 calories. They can be a protein (powder, meat, fish…), a fruit (most fruits are 50-120 calories) or unlimited non-starchy vegetables. Because of the very low sugar/starch and high fiber in vegetables, it is unlikely you would eat too many if you eat them raw or steamed with no added fat. A small amount of beans with no added fat is also OK for variety. Remember the lower your calorie intake in a 24-hour period, especially during daylight hours, the faster you will lose body fat if you follow all the other steps. For the most rapid fat loss, follow the guidelines set forth for SuperHighway eating and always shoot for a minimum of 300 but no more than 800 calories per day.

Fresh fruits and vegetables make perfect TurboCharged meals. They are high in water, vitamins, minerals and fiber while containing natural sugars that will satisfy your sweet tooth. The crunchiness will keep your jaws happy. The best benefit is that they are also low in calories so you can really eat a lot. For comparison, you'd have to consume a huge amount of vegetables in one sitting to come anywhere close to that 440-calorie slice of cheesecake or chocolate cake.

Cucumbers, radishes, zucchini, celery, red and green peppers, cauliflower, mushrooms and broccoli are all less than 10 calories an ounce. They also contain lots of water. As we have discussed, most hunger pangs are really indications of thirst. Reaching for fruits and vegetables along with 16 to 32 ounces of water will do wonders to rev up your TurboCharger. Fruits, which are unnecessarily limited in so many diets, provide great satisfaction due to their higher moisture and sugar content. Unlike a piece of candy or those slices of cake we just talked about, fruit, with its ability to "fill us up," its natural vitamins and minerals, along with its sweetness, is a real bargain.

As you look through the list below, keep in mind how unsatisfied you might feel if you could only eat 2/5 of an ounce of potato chips (that's about 3-5 chips!), not even 1/3 of a very small muffin, less than a quarter of the average commercial bakery cookie, a small quarter-cup of cereal with milk, or a couple of spoonfuls of ice cream. Each of these would be about 100 calories and they are carbohydrate and fat combinations that would most likely spike insulin levels, totally defeating all of your progress.

DON'T BE FOOLED…by those new "100-Calorie Packages" of goldfish, pretzels, cookies or anything else commercially packaged and advertised. As we have mentioned before, manufacturers and advertisers alike are tuning into the concept of 100-calorie meals and trying to confuse you while working this to their dollar advantage. These packaged foods are harmful because their carbohydrate and fat combinations, along with their very low moisture content, will result in overconsumption. This will immediately spike your insulin levels, once again putting your body back on the fat-storage, depression-oriented roller coaster. One-hundred-calorie prepackaged foods have no place in TurboCharged bodies—even if they claim to be sugar-free or fat-free. Regardless of their claims, they will slow or stop your progress, stripping you of your championship finish. Be wise, and choose your TurboCharged mini-meals from the extensive list that follows.

100-CALORIE (or less) TURBOCHARGED FOODS…In No Particular Order

Note #1: This list doesn't include all the cookies, cakes, etc. that are currently being packaged as "Only 100" calories. If you eat these the sugar load they produce will immediately halt TurboCharging while re-triggering moodiness and stress.

Note #2: This list is provided as a reference for your SuperHighway days. At other times—taking the Expressway

or once you've reached Cruise Control—after drinking up plenty of water and following the TurboCharged steps, feel free to eat as much as you want. Be sure to follow the nutrient separation and food guidelines that we recommend.

15 thin fillets of anchovies
1 large apple
1 large hard-boiled egg sliced and sprinkled with cumin, celery seed or nutmeg
3 ounces of deli turkey spread with Dijon mustard and rolled in romaine or Boston lettuce leaves
5 fresh apricots
1 large artichoke
30 spears of steamed, fresh asparagus
¼ avocado
½ cup of edamame
¾ cup mango tossed with limejuice and red pepper flakes
2 slices of broiled bacon (hopefully nitrate-free)
1 large banana
¾ cup lima beans, cooked
4 cups string beans
1 slice of corned beef
1 cup jicama sticks with 2 tablespoons of hummus for dipping
1 slice of lean loin of beef
1 lean rib of beef
½ can of beer
4 cooked, fresh beets
40 blackberries
1 cup of blueberries
1 3oz piece of bluefish, baked or broiled
A small wedge of Brie
3 hearty stalks of broccoli
1-½ cups cooked Brussels sprouts
1 medium baked potato cooked (pierce and microwave for 4 minutes) topped with salsa

3 cups of fresh cabbage (packed)

1 wedge Camembert cheese

½ cantaloupe

2 cups of fresh or steamed carrots

3 cups of fresh or steamed cauliflower

6 cups of celery

A 1-inch cube of cheddar

1 cup of cherries

A slice of broiled or roasted chicken

6 clams

A small cappuccino with half-and-half

1 cup corn

½ cup fresh crabmeat

2 tbsp. cream cheese spread onto celery sticks

2 tablespoons of cream cheese with a little onion powder & pepper and unlimited celery sticks

3 large cucumbers

4 dates

2 dates with a little fresh peanut butter inside them (after removing the pit!)

½ breast or a thigh of duck

1 egg anyway you want it

Figs, fresh (3) or dried (2)

Fish – a slice of flounder, halibut, haddock, etc.

1 frankfurter (if you must!)

1 cup fresh fruit salad

½ cup gefilte fish

1 slice of goose

1 grapefruit

A large bunch of grapes, about 40 juicy ones

1 slice of ham

1 very small hamburger patty

¾ honeydew melon

1½ cups kale

1 lamb rib chop

7 big leeks
2 heads lettuce—eat as much as you want…just skip the oily dressing
2/3 cup lobster
1 slice of any luncheon meat (they are all about the same)
10 fresh mushrooms
8 mussels
25 pieces of okra
16 extra large olives—green & ripe
2/3 of a bowl onion soup
A juicy fresh orange
2/3 cup of fresh parsnips
2 peaches
20 roasted peanuts
1 large pear
¾ cup green peas
½ cup split pea soup
5 green peppers
6 dill pickles
3 sweet pickles—check the label for sugar!
2 fresh pineapple slices
4 fresh plums
½ broiled pork chop
1 medium baked potato (sans the butter or sour cream—remember, no fats and carbs!)
4 dried prunes
40 radishes
A small handful of raisins
1 glass of red wine
6 cups of rhubarb
Roquefort cheese - one wedge
A piece of salmon, swordfish or tuna about the size of a deck of cards
5 sardines
15 shrimp

2 cups of cooked spinach
3 cups of squash-boiled
2 cups of fresh strawberries
½ sweet potato
2 large tangerines
3 juicy tomatoes
¼ cup tuna fish
1 slice of turkey
2 cups of turnip
1 cup vegetable soup
10 walnut halves
4 bunches of watercress
1 glass of white wine

CALORIES IN FRUIT: fresh fruit, unsweetened, as offered by Nature

Note: 100 grams equals a little less than 4 ounces

Eat in unlimited quantities except during your SuperHighway days.

Apples (all varieties)	1 medium	65
	1 large	100
Apricots	1 large	20
Avocado	1 medium	255
Banana	1 large	100
Blueberries	1 cup	50
Blackberries	1 cup	50
Cantaloupe	1 cubed cup	40
Cherries	1 medium	5
Coconut	4 ounces	270
Cranberries	1/2 cup	20
Cumquats	6 large	50
Dates	3	160

Figs	1 medium	50
Fruit Salad (fresh)	1 cup mixed	120
Grapefruit	1 medium	20
Grapes	1 large bunch	310
Kiwi	1 medium	40
Lemon	1 medium	25
Lime	1 small	10
Lychees	1 medium	10
Mango	1 medium	100
Nectarine	1 medium	30
Olives (any kind)	1 medium	10
Oranges	1 medium	80
Clementines or Mandarin		35
Papaya	1 small or 1/2 large	80
Passion fruit	1 medium	15
Peaches	1 medium	40
Pears	1 medium	70
Pineapple	1 cup cubed	55
Plums	1 medium	35
Pomegranate	1/2 medium	75
Raspberries	6 ounces/1 cup	25
Rhubarb	1 cup cubed	25
Strawberries	1 large	10
Tangerine	1 small	35
Tomato	1 medium	20
Watermelon	1 thick slice	70

Calories in Fresh Vegetables:

Alfalfa Sprouts	100 grams	30
Artichoke	medium	20
Asparagus	6 spears	20
Bamboo Shoots	8 ounces	20
Beans (string)	1 cup	30

Lima beans	8 ounces	20
Kidney beans	8 ounces	100
Chick Peas (cooked)	100 grams	100
Lentils	100 grams	70
Beets	4 oz.	30
Broccoli	1 cup	20
Brussels Sprouts	4 sprouts	25
Cabbage	1 cup	20
Carrots	1 medium	35
Celery	1 stick	5
Chard, Swiss	1 cup	7
Collards	1 cup	11
Corn	1 cob	60
	1/2 cup	50
Cucumber	1 medium	10
Dill Pickles	1 large	10
Eggplant	1 cup	35
fried in oil	100 grams	140
Kale	1 cup	50
Kohlrabi	100 grams	35
Lettuce (any kind)	don't even bother counting it is so low! Eat up!	
Leeks	1 whole	10
Mung Beans (sprouts)	1 cup	20
Mushrooms	lots	30
Okra	10 pods	25
Onions	1 medium	30
Parsley	bunches	4
Parsnip	100 grams	50
Peas- (Green)	1 cup	134
(Snow)	10 pods	10
(Snap)	10 pods	10
Potatoes (Baked)	1 medium	175
Pumpkin	100 grams	120

Sauerkraut	1 cup	50
Shallots	3	5
Spinach	100 grams	15
Squash	100 grams	25
Sweet Potato	medium	103
Taro	100 grams	110
Tomato (Raw)	1 medium	20
Cherry Tomato	1	4
Turnip	100 grams	15
Watercress	a bunch	20
Yam	1 cup steamed	119
Zucchini	1 medium	30

TurboCharged Fast Foods

When beginning the TurboCharged program, many initially stall because they are so used to complicated regimens and recipes. To help get you moving, here are some sample "recipes" of delicious "fast" foods you can enjoy.

- Buy frozen or canned beans and/or vegetables; empty them into a strainer and rinse to eliminate sugary/salty juice. Season with pepper or spices of your choice. Eat immediately or refrigerate and eat within two days. Note: Well-rinsed canned hearts of palm are delicious!

- The most obvious fast food is any amount of cut-up, fresh fruits or vegetables. You can add a spicy sour cream or softened cream cheese dip used very sparingly. This will add great satisfaction along with some fat and protein for hormone production. The TurboCharged rule is the cheese/dip should be 10% or less of the total volume.

- Low carbohydrate tortillas made with soy or flax seed (3-5 net carbohydrate grams per serving*) with melted cheese, meat, fish, eggs or tofu. Feel free to spice it up (sans salt) or add chopped vegetables such as chives or other fresh herbs, onions, garlic, avocado, olives, etc. These tortillas may take you briefly out of fat-burning mode. However, this little variety, once or twice a week, might be just what you need to keep going strong. *To calculate net carbohydrate number: Carbohydrate – Fiber = Net Carbohydrates

- Cook up some eggs, ground beef, pork, chicken or tofu. Add seasonings of your choice if you desire.

- Try lettuce leaves in place of bread to make a healthy "sandwich" with a slice of your favorite cheese, meat, fish or tofu.

- Mash up some avocado and make your own "guacamole" and wrap it in lettuce.

- Roll up cheese in any cold cut meat and enjoy.

- Cut up several large, sweet apples and after eating a few slices, if you want more, have a handful of the raw nut of your choice.

- Eat a few slices of apple along with a small handful of pumpkin seeds, including the shells.

- Chop up an avocado and mix with some sugar-free salsa, a squeeze of lime and some fresh chopped cilantro. Use romaine or endive lettuce leaves or slices of a hearty pepper instead of chips for dipping.

- Open a can of tuna or salmon. Chop in some onion or celery, add a little olive oil to taste, and enjoy.

- A cup of cappuccino, coffee or tea (regular or decaf) with half-and-half (try to make sure to add no more than two tablespoons of cream which equals 35 calories).

- A handful of raw walnuts, almonds, macadamias or pecans.

- A frozen banana. Peel a few, wrap or put in a plastic bag and put in your freezer. Once frozen, remove and put a napkin around base to hold. It is just like an ice cream. Kids love these. Introduce them to babies as young as 10 months old, and you'll be creating a healthy palate.

- Scrambled eggs.

- A slice or two of organic cheese of choice. Raw cheese is best if you can find it.

- 8-10 Clementines.

- Two or three organic Mejool dates stuffed with organic no-salt nut butter.

- An apple sliced and dunked lightly into Glaser Farms Organic Raw Italian Almond Butter (glaserorganic-farms.com) Expensive nut butters…but off-the-charts delicious!

- Frozen grapes. Rinse. Pick them off the stem. Load them into a freezer bag or container. Freeze for about 8 hours. Enjoy!

A Few Notes:

With personal experimentation supported by research, we have observed that periods of eating just fruits and vegetables will increase protein efficiency. Protein is recycled in the body, so if you aim to eat protein at just one meal daily, when you do eat protein, your body will utilize it much more efficiently. Further, with the naturally lower-calorie meals, high water content and truly natural sugar that fruits and vegetables provide throughout the day, your insulin sensitivity will greatly improve. The benefit of this to your body: it will no longer readily store carbohydrates as fat.

If you use whole foods instead of shakes, just make sure that at least one meal out of every three contains about 20-25 grams of protein in any form. Good protein sources are any kind of meat, fish, eggs and tofu without any hormones or additives. For those with cardiovascular issues, the literature is still divided on cheese, so we recommend that you limit your cheese consumption to no more than three or four times per week. Bacon? Keep it as a Sunday treat. Also, yogurt and other milk and dairy products are not part of a TurboCharged diet. Although yogurt may be a good food, it contains too much sugar and cannot be part of the TurboCharged fat reduction plan. Save the yogurt for a treat meal once you have reached your goal, and even then only eat the Greek unsweetened, whole fat kind—not 0% which is too high in sugar.

Beginning TurboChargers may wonder why they are not hungry even when at times they are eating so little. The answer is this: We maintain our muscle mass by walking and doing our one-minute workouts while also keeping our tanks filled to the brim with plenty of water or other non-caloric, unsweetened fluids and eating tasty TurboCharged foods. The brain, subsequently, supports our goal of a sleek, lean and healthy body and is content consuming our body fat. Cooperate with this lack of hunger and enjoy it without worrying about food.

Success in any endeavor is not about perfection. Success is all about consistency. The TurboCharged program is no different. The more consistent you are with all the steps over a week, month or year, the better your results will be. The steps are designed to be so simple that anyone can fit them into their life no matter how hectic it is. When thinking about your day, you need to put together a plan for your eating and mini-sessions that you can follow consistently. Planning to do a strict SuperHighway trip for too long a time period (especially longer than 10 consecutive days) is a recipe for failure. Sometimes even 10 days is too long, so try a shorter time period of every 3-5 days maximum as your schedule allows, but stick with all the other steps and meal guidelines the rest of the time. Have a free TurboCharged Expressway day then get back onto the SuperHighway until you reach your goal. You will cross the finish line in record time!

Watch Out for False-Urge Roadblocks

Be forewarned that when you first begin you may feel deprived and unfulfilled because food has been a major time-filler, replacing the fun things you enjoyed as a child and teenager. Fun is severely lacking in most of our lives. Watching reality TV or sitcoms might seem like fun ways to pass time, but these are not productive or fulfilling activities. Meals filled with every kind of delicious food may seem quite enjoyable while you are eating them, but they are not fulfilling because they don't support your goal. There is no substitute for adding some fun new activities in your life and using them to reclaim your vitality and passion.

Reading a book, learning something new, becoming skilled in a sport, language, musical instrument or any intellectual activity may not initially be as appealing as sitting on a couch, watching DVDs and devouring a half gallon of ice cream after that large pizza. However, productive actions fulfill us far more and lead to rejuvenation from the inside out. It is critical to relocate and revive the activities that make us feel good after doing them, not merely during the activity. Use your mind and body and be creative. Think about new things to do to fill your time with activities, projects and new accomplishments that will make you feel truly good from the inside out.

It is also important to remember that most of us are addicted to constantly eating foods that produce a sugar rush. If the daily challenges of life are weighing you down and your spirits feel like they are dipping, binge on fresh fruits. See how many you can eat. Load up! Have plenty of fruits on hand at all times. If you still need "something" you might grab a handful of raw, unsalted nuts to chew very slowly and thoughtfully. Within a week or less, your blood sugar levels will be much more stabilized and you will be able to go much longer on very little food while relying more and more on your body fat. Being TurboCharged will significantly change your life and health. Reread this paragraph, memorize it and you will be well on your way to the Winner's Circle!

What do I do if I start to stall?

In any eating plan, there can come a time when the body seems to plateau at a particular weight. While we have never witnessed anyone lose 30 pounds of fat in 30 days, 20-25 pounds is quite common. Dian lost 20 pounds in 24 days exactly. Most people start out with about 20-40 pounds of excess body fat to get rid of before they are at the ideal state of "lean." During the first week the results are dramatic and usually reach 1-2 pounds of body fat (based on a Tanita scale) per day. Some continue this for weeks. That said, TurboChargers generally do well 20-25 days a month by strictly following the program. When combining foods, we recommend the 90/10% rule to be an "eyeball" rule. In this book we talk about volume of food while providing calorie information because this makes it more "accountable" for some. If you are following all the steps but getting less-than-satisfying results, you are 1) not eating enough fruits and vegetables during the day and/or 2) consuming excess fat/carbohydrate combinations and/or 3) you are neglecting to walk and aren't being active enough in other areas and/ or 4) you are ignoring the importance of your mini-weight workout routines. If you are not seeing enough progress, you are not following one or more of the steps. Remember, this is a program where each step is like a part working together with others to create a fully functioning engine. Make the program as pleasurable as possible but give yourself the option of being very rigorous for extra-exciting results whenever your schedule allows.

Another problem some TurboChargers encounter is that they are making great progress getting trim but still are shy of "sleek and lean." This is because they are only doing the mini-routines 2-3 times per day. This will usually work for weeks or even months. Some people then stall. If this is you, move up the "weight levels" and go to 4-5 times per day. What are "light weights" for two weeks may be too light during weeks three or four. Adding a little more weight every couple of weeks will still be "light" because you will be getting much stronger, and this will add the muscle that increases your metabolism. It will actually make you naturally desire smaller portions of food.

TurboChargers will sometimes try a fruit day with little or no protein/fat coupled with a higher frequency of light weights. They may even walk intermittently for a total of one to two hours per day and take many relaxing fluid breaks. This results in a very dramatic and visible reduction of both visceral and subcutaneous body fat. The next day, they add whatever vegetables they want and they see the same results. So TurboChargers learn that they can always have the dramatic reductions they desire by reverting to this 1-2 day regimen. TurboChargers always comment on how absolutely fantastic they feel after both days. The challenge is then to be "conscious" of the way you are doing all of the steps. With a good body-fat scale, TurboChargers can see how well they are following the plan.

The Big Question

Cheating? Cheating is not counting certain foods in your total calorie count while doing a SuperHighway run. It is pretending something doesn't count or that something can be substituted without consequence. It is eating a cellophane-wrapped "100 Calorie" carbohydrate/fat snack or a candy bar. You get the picture. Let us tell you loud and clear: Anything outside of the TurboCharged food list will slow you down. The only person hurt when cheating is YOU.

Here are some things you might want to think about to stay on the "straight and narrow" roadway (which is actually quite wide!) without losing traction:

- Insulin-producing foods cause a great deal of water retention. Just one day eating these foods may cause a weight increase of 3-5 pounds and this can happen on any diet.

- Calorie-dense foods will stimulate memories in your brain of all the "pleasures" of those foods and they will stimulate your appetite until you can't get enough. Your body fat will return and sometimes more. This will be very discouraging, as you probably already know.

- Eating your old way will return body fat rapidly.

- "Starting all over again" is old news and is what happens to you on regular "weight loss" diets. TurboCharged is holistic and gives you all the tools needed to end past patterns and reach the goal of a sleek physique with lean muscles for life.

- You will always get excited by the idea of cutting loose with friends or family and eating a buffet of tantalizing foods without concern. But you should know by now that the next day or two you will be disappointed by your decision to interrupt your road trip to success. You will not think the two hours of hedonism was worth the after effects.

- When you are thinking about eating any dessert besides fresh, delicious, sweet fruits, remember this: STRESSED spelled backwards is DESSERTS!

You are in the driver's seat. If you fishtail or start to spin out, get yourself straight and keep going back in the right direction. Stay away from the foods, naysayers or anything taking you from your destination of Fabulosity! Take a walk, visualize your buff TurboCharged body, grab a big drink of water or other noncaloric beverage and fill up, brush your teeth and rinse vigorously with mouthwash, then drop down and do some push-ups, squats or lunges! You are in control.

What if I make a mistake or blow an entire day?

"So what?" we say. TurboChargers get back in the driver's seat and leave the drama in Hollywood. We make a commitment and stick with it until we are walking around in our sleek, lean, fabulous, healthy, enviable, awe-inspiring bodies. If you blow a meal or a whole day, so what? You are on a mission. Pull over, fill up your tank and get back on the track. Do a few extra one-minute weight routines to get back in touch with your muscles, body and spirit. Take a couple of extra 10-minute walks. Do not become discouraged and do not stop until you can do at least 10 days straight eating just TurboCharged food choices in any quantity you desire. Once you finish a 10-day period, the value of becoming TurboCharged will be obvious. We know you can do this. Just do it! You belong in the Winner's Circle.

TurboCharging is a program for life. It is not a diet. It is a new way of living healthfully. As such, there is no such thing as mistakes or cheating. Rather, we view these instances as lessons we may need to get refocused. Embrace the moment and yourself—then remember you are on a mission.

A First Time Loser Since TurboCharging

At age 50, Bob Aldrich decided to try TurboCharged for his first-ever weight-loss program. He's a big guy at 6'2". He had weighed 190 pounds for most of his adult life with a body-fat reading of 23.5%. With TurboCharged, he lost 25 pounds to weigh in at a solid 165 pounds with 11.4% body fat. Best of all, his blood pressure went from 135 over 85 to 110 over 70, and he lost four inches from his waist.

"The TurboCharged regimen enabled my body to burn its own fat, as the program promises it will. I easily lost one to two pounds a day," says Bob. "I was never hungry and had energy to spare. Until I started talking to experienced dieters, I thought all weight-loss programs were this easy. Boy, was I mistaken."

A wine aficionado, Bob frequently attended events with 10-course dinners, where he admits to consuming up to 6,000 calories in one meal. Also, as a bread lover all of his life, he often ate six pieces of bread with olive oil or butter in addition to a main menu. With TurboCharged, Bob committed to take the SuperHighway approach. He maintained a 300 to 500-calorie food intake of strictly TurboCharged food choices until he reached his goal with a few Expressway days thrown in. He now finds that should a craving strike one piece of bread now satisfies the urge, and fresh or canned tuna, salmon or sardines along with huge bowls of fresh fruit are his new daily indulgences.

"I'm a very busy guy. What makes TurboCharged work for my lifestyle are the simple one-minute muscle-building routines scheduled throughout the day, plus walking after dinner. I now know that this charges the metabolism to burn fat for fuel," says Bob. "On any diet, if you increase your activity level and limit the starches and calories, you will lose weight until you go off the diet. TurboCharged, though, is different. You do not regain, period. It is a big breakthrough because it is a new way of living and thinking about food."

Now let's move on to Step #8. We will learn how TurboChargers visualize the rewards of being a champion.

Step #8
"Seeing" the Prize

Stress, as we discussed a bit earlier, is counterproductive to TurboCharging. Sleep, rest and relaxation are essential for reaching the ultimate body you desire. To really get sleek and lean fast, you will want to get a good night's rest. Lots of fat burning occurs when you are sleeping. During the day, you will be supporting your fat burning (and subsequent muscle retention) by incorporating mini-minutes of rest into your life. Of course, if your life is extremely busy and filled with stressful demands and time commitments, feel free to skip this step. Only kidding! You need rest and relaxation all the more.

TurboChargers in high fat-burning mode sleep as much as possible. Body fat is naturally being burned for energy during sleep because you aren't eating; yet the body must continue fulfilling its countless essential functions. Eight-plus hours are optimal for fat burning. Hit the sack early and you will TurboCharge more quickly. People who get five or less hours of sleep per night are 55% more likely to be obese than those who log eight hours plus nightly. Sleep deprivation seems to increase cravings for high fat-carb foods. Try this recipe for a good night's sleep: Start with a warm cup of chamomile tea in the early evening or some other non-caffeinated tea of your choice. Put on some comfy bedtime clothes. Cuddle with your children, if you have them and they'll let you, and talk. Read a good bedtime story with a non-stressful theme. Turn off the lights and say goodbye to the fridge until the morning. Skip the TV at night. A study from the Harvard School of Public Health in Boston reports that for every two hours of TV you watch daily, your risk for obesity rises 23%. Besides the inactivity factor, there is the added temptation from food commercials, purposefully designed by experts, to derail your best intentions when you are tired and most vulnerable. Nighttime TV is loaded with hunger-inspiring messages that you don't need trying to invade your peaceful dreams of a lean TurboCharged physique.

Daytime Rest

Not all of us can afford the luxury of a daytime nap, which would assist in daytime fat burning. That said, regardless of where you are—work, home, on vacation, driving across country, traveling by plane or train—you can take a *minute* to relax and consequently accelerate your progress.

The same will and determination you use to get through your busy day can be applied to reach fully TurboCharged status. You have the power to focus your mind, to practice creative visualization and meditation, so that you can succeed not just today, but for however long it takes you to reach your personal finish line to claim the reward of the healthy, lean body you were meant to have.

Many studies acknowledge and confirm the benefits of this vital daytime relaxation step. We, Dian and Tom, have spent over 40 collective years studying all forms of meditation, prayer, hypnosis and creative visualization. TurboChargers know this step cannot be overlooked. Despite how driven and committed you are to your life and work, you cannot be as effective if you are constantly experiencing stress. Stress is good and even healthy if summoned occasionally to increase our reserves, effort and stamina. But non-stop stress is debilitating. It lowers immunity and severely hampers hormonal functioning and healing. Stress is driven by worry, guilt and fear: the fear of failure, falling behind, not doing enough and not being good enough. These worries, fears, insecurities and the resulting stress cause us to react in the moment and this often makes us forget our long-term goals and needs. When left unchecked, this stress will cause us to react automatically and unconsciously to external stimuli. This means we might eat for no other reason but that we no longer feel in full control.

With this step, you are going to learn to relax for a lifetime of TurboCharged success.

Seeing the Reward

It is never too late to begin practicing meditation or incorporating visualization into your life. Meditation, prayer, visualization, self-hypnosis, creative visualization all serve the same purpose. They are an effective time-out from the events of the day: the boss at work, the screaming client, the person driving 20 miles an hour in the 45-mile-an-hour zone, the needs and demands of your children. Simply put: Time out from life in general.

How you choose to relax is your option. However, regular one-minute intervals (at least) represent a critical step to TurboCharging. The time you spend relaxing is not actually as important as the fact that you simply just stop and do it. Even if it is only for a minute, the effect of simply stopping any thought or activity to breathe deeply can do wonders for stress levels, health, well-being—and fat burning too!

There are two simple and interchangeable ways you can practice this relaxation step. Do one, the other or both. But choose and do it.

Meditative Breathing: This is a very simple strategy. Whether it is screaming kids, work stress, or anything else, you can find a quiet place and a minute to relax. A shut door closing off the world or a bathroom stall works just fine. Pulling over to the side of the road in a traffic jam can work too. Stop and close your eyes. Take a deep breath in through your nose and release while trying to do your best Darth Vader imitation. Clear your mind by simply focusing on breathing in and breathing out. Think or recite "breathe in, breathe out" if needed to keep other thoughts at bay. Aim for 10 deep breaths minimum, more if time allows. Simply concentrate on: Breathe in, breathe out.

Creative Visualization: Visualization is a highly effective technique that uses your ever-present imagination to your advantage. Too often, at some age, we forget the power of the imagination that allowed us to stay occupied as children for hours on end. Athletes use visualization. Hockey phenomenon Wayne Gretzky practiced creative visualization. When asked what made him superior to other players he commented, "A good player plays where the puck is; a great player to where it is going to be." Broadway stars overcome fears by visualizing the applause at the end of their spectacular performance. A baseball player might imagine the exhilaration of running the bases after hitting a home run.

Anyone can visualize a goal. Maybe you can summon up a good image of the body you want. "See" the new look you will have when you reach your goal. Details count. So again, you want to find a quiet place, if even only for a moment, and imagine. Imagine the thrill of slipping into a bathing suit and feeling like you fit in it or that you have regained some of your youth or that your muscles are sleek and taut. You notice those muscles: the curves on your arms, the tightness in your abdominal muscles. The fat is long gone. You have a trim and tight waist. You can wear whatever you want. Imagine yourself smiling every time you see your new reflection in a mirror.

Using your imagination in a positive way is very constructive. You are giving your mind the blueprint, much like an architect provides to the builder, to see exactly what the finished building will look like.

Visualizing and meditation are essential to making your dreams reality.

Stress is the most significant element that causes the brain to go into a defensive mode. As you now know, this causes the dire consequence of breaking down vital muscle tissue to release sugar for additional energy. The massive imbalance this stress creates is a formidable opponent that can bring great hunger along for the ride with fear and anxiety as well. Rest and relaxation, even in one-minute intervals a few times each day, are proven to have a huge impact in keeping your body fully TurboCharged.

If for any reason you are really struggling with visualizing and cannot imagine yourself lean and healthy, feel free to borrow a picture of someone else's body that you admire and attach your face. Do whatever is necessary to get your mind thinking positively. This isn't flaky. It is science. You are marshalling your super-powerful subconscious mind to unlock your inner strength. This step will TurboCharge you!

Affirmations to Support Your Meditation and Visualization

Affirmations support meditation and visualization. An affirmation statement is ideally 20 words or less. The brevity is important, because if it gets too long, it is simply too hard to remember, and you do want to remember it.

To be effective, your affirmation must clearly define your present goals and philosophy. It is a flexible statement that you may want to refine as you go along and are reaching your objectives. Writing a personal affirmation statement is not a test. Feel free to have more than one. It is a support tool that you can post on your refrigerator, desktop and bathroom mirror or wherever you might see it often. The more often you think about your affirmation, the better. It is a gentle reminder that you are working to be the best you can be.

Here are a few samples of our favorites:

- Every day in every way I am getting better and better!

- I choose healthy foods, fun activities, and surround myself with good friends who support my success.

- I laugh as often as possible and remember that a smile counts as facial activity!

- I am getting healthier and healthier every day!

- I am getting leaner, stronger and sexier with each step I take!

- Today I will do what I can, and tomorrow I will be able to do even more.

° Each choice I make supports my TurboCharged body.

° I deserve to be slender and healthy. God intended this to be so.

° The Universe supports my goal of a lean, healthy body.

° No matter what challenges I face, I am forever committed to my healthy, lean body.

° I embrace my perfect body as I get more attractive, leaner and healthier every day.

Looking 10 Years Younger Thanks to TurboCharged

Bonnie Watkins is a 57-year-old wife and mother with a high-stress administrative job. Bonnie reports that she has "personalized" the TurboCharged program to achieve optimum results. Whatever she did, one can't argue with her remarkable success. She's lost 25 pounds, going from 145 to 120 pounds, an ideal weight for her 5'5" frame. She now has a body-fat reading of 20%. Her dress size has dropped from size 8 to size 4.

"In terms of energy and general joie de vivre, I feel like I did when I was 40," says Bonnie. "I honestly turned the clock back a decade. The TurboCharged program is the menu for the rest of my life." Bonnie achieved her results in less than two months, which is typical for TurboCharged followers. She's amazed by her great results and how much she enjoys the program itself. She says that TurboCharged has been her "dream come true."

"TurboCharged is the easiest, healthiest and fastest fat-loss program ever," says Bonnie. "I am now at the weight I want to be, and I will eat the TurboCharged way for life." Her typical TurboCharged meals include a bowl of fruit and a hard-boiled egg for breakfast, a banana and an apple for lunch, and roasted vegetables for dinner. "I find it simple as well as satisfying to eat as many vegetables as I want for dinner. Sometimes I follow the TurboCharged '90-10' rule and add a small piece of fish, chicken or tofu."

Bonnie adds, "My husband, Bruce, joined me on this adventure. He did not always follow the program steps as strictly as he could have, but was always careful to avoid any insulin-triggering foods. He, too, had excellent results."

Maintaining Your TurboCharged Body: Just Hit Cruise Control

In the near future, if you have chosen to follow the program faithfully, the day will come when you are strong and fully TurboCharged. Excess body fat is a memory. **You become a highly efficient hybrid vehicle. Your body easily derives its energy needs from the Turbocharged foods, constantly and effortlessly switching between sugar, proteins and fat.** Your moods are consistent and improved. After trying so hard in the past, you never knew it would be so easy to reach your goal. You now realize that it wasn't you; it was the poor advice you received. You always had the determination. You just needed the right information and tools.

When TurboChargers reach their goal, they hit the cruise control button. When you get to your ideal, sleek, lean and high-performance body, you will be well-tuned. You will have a new understanding of how your body works and what makes it feel and perform best. You will automatically know how much you need to eat in order to keep things in shape and running smoothly.

Cruise control is easy. There is no need to constantly watch the speedometer. You have things under control. You will keep doing all the Steps in regular intervals. You will continue to put the correct fuel in your body. You will continue to eat the TurboCharged way. You will just eat more. At this point, you will instinctively know the right amount.

One key point worth mentioning here is that people are into rituals as to set times they "should" eat versus eating when truly hungry, and, worse, they are dedicated to meal "sizes" thinking they won't be full unless their plate is. This is a sad cultural phenomenon. When fully TurboCharged, people lose feelings of hunger for excess food that is above and beyond their normal metabolic requirements. They are enjoying the vitality and energy that results from sourcing any excess body fat for energy needs. What this means to you is that when we tell you to not insist on "portion" sizes, we are saying two things: "Don't eat small or limited portions" and "Don't eat if you are not really hungry."

"Portion size" and set meal times are common roadblocks inherent to most weight-loss programs. When your body gets fully TurboCharged, "portion size" resolves itself because we are satisfied with less and less food. We only eat when we are hungry, because excess body fat has become our primary source of energy. We explain to new TurboChargers that when they feel full and satisfied on a piece of chicken or beef or two pieces of fruit, they should not keep eating in order to match their previous portion ideals. Go along with this new and exciting information your body is giving you! Your TurboCharger is kicking in and your body is feeling satisfied by using your excess body fat for energy. Go with it and don't fight it by adding more food than needed just to satisfy an old memory of "portion size." Instead, get out and walk, do your weight routines, fill up your tank with that perfect fluid—water—and FORGET ABOUT FOOD!

Yes, this often means that for days at a time you might be eating very, very little because your body is happily using your body fat. That is the function and beauty of TurboCharging. But it is a very difficult concept to internalize as we've been told so many times throughout our lives that "we need to eat." Until you experience this, it is truly hard to fathom. Yet every TurboCharger reports this same phenomenon!

Of course, there are days when we TurboChargers are just hungrier—plain and simple. On those days we continue to follow our energizing steps of drinking plenty of non-caloric fluids, walking and doing the one-minute weight-resistance routines. We eat plenty. Sometimes even a few thousand calories, but we stick with TurboCharged foods. Tom has been known to eat a pound of steak whereas Dian can easily eat a pound of nuts!

The power of the program is this: Once you are TurboCharged, your hunger naturally adjusts to a perfect level to maintain a lean, healthy body. The number of calories you consume becomes inconsequential as long as you stick with TurboCharged foods and continue doing all the other steps.

So remember: If you aren't hungry, don't eat; and when you are hungry, don't worry about the portion size. If the portion that satisfies you is large or if it seems miniscule, go with your body's inherent intelligence and be assured that it is doing just fine feeding itself all the energy it needs from any excess body fat you have. The minute you are truly lean, your hunger and appetite will adjust accordingly, but you will likely be surprised to find that it is shockingly...well, much different than you might ever have believed if you hadn't experienced the TurboCharged program.

When you become lean and healthy, you will know when you can eat some of your old favorites. Until you are at your ideal body-fat percentage and at the appropriate weight according to the height listed in the chart provided earlier, we recommend you wait on those old favorites until you are truly TurboCharged.

Old Favorites

Let's address that "old favorites" part. Our body becomes acutely sensitive when we restrict foods to lose a great deal of body fat. Going back to large regular meals, especially if they include carbohydrates in the form of pizza, pasta, grains, rice, breads, cookies, cakes and pastries, for example, will remind the brain of all those calorie-loaded tastes. You will be overwhelmed by a lifetime of stored associations involving rich "comfort" foods along with in-grained (no pun intended) feelings of reward and satisfaction. The body will utilize these calories very efficiently, meaning it will put back the body fat you just lost very rapidly, especially if you eat too much of this junk too many days in a row. Higher insulin levels from these non-turbocharged foods will also cause a major psych-out as they will increase water retention and 3-5 extra pounds will appear within hours. Mood swings will strike. One or two consecutive full days of non-turbocharged foods will take 3-4 days of strict TurboCharged eating to get your body back into fat-burning mode. It will trigger your body to once again rely on sugar vs. excess body fat for its energy requirements. This will be discouraging and delay progress. So what's our advice? Never forget the goal. We say nothing tastes better than living a long healthy life in a lean, fabulous-looking, relaxed body!

Once you develop the habit of TurboCharging every time you notice your hunger, it is very hard to really want food that might not keep you burning fat. TurboCharging causes muscles to rebound. It will keep your body using your excess body fat for fuel instead of relying on fat-storing sugar. TurboCharging keeps you relaxed. TurboCharged provides the steps to make sure you are eating only when you are truly hungry and not eating just because you are bored, frustrated, celebrating or any other reason you may have used in the past.

You may occasionally decide, maybe once a week, to stray from TurboCharging by eating crackers with some cheese, guacamole with chips or having a turkey sandwich with lettuce and tomato on whole-grain bread or some other non-turbocharged food. Once you have reached your goal, if this is what you want to do once in a while, that's your choice. The sugar in the cracker, chip or bread may temporarily stop your fat burning, but there is no reason to start a bunch of drama worthy of an Oscar! Instead, enjoy your choice; knowing that for your health, you can continue to follow the TurboCharged steps for life. This is what will keep you burning fat as you cruise around in the body you have desired for so long. You now have a new understanding and appreciation for how your body works best. If you are at your goal, that occasional meal will not hurt your ultimate health or add fat onto your body. It may simply trigger your body to derive energy from glucose instead of body fat and dietary fat for a few hours, assuming you get right back on course.

We prefer to maintain our physiques with unlimited amounts of TurboCharged foods. Just knowing we will never again experience indigestion is inspiring enough! Occasionally we might grab that chip with guacamole or really hot toasty bread in a great restaurant, but for the most part we have found that we have genuinely altered our cravings, taste buds, and food preferences. Given a choice, a large fresh fruit salad really is much more sweet, satiating and appealing than any cookie we can think of, except maybe the ones our mom makes, but even she knows we need the healthiest version possible!

You, too, may be surprised. But don't be. Your body and heart will always steer you in a direction of health and well-being if you listen closely and allow their innate wisdom to help you reach your goals.

You can do it. We know you can. Today you have in your hands all the knowledge and tools necessary for your success. All you need to add is a little determination to get the chemical reaction brewing.

Make your new mantra: I can be TurboCharged, I know I can. I will keep going and never, ever stop. Refuse to listen to excuses. Remove yourself from naysayers that want you to "pull over" because they don't have your determination and willpower. Block out any distractions. Forget past failures, false starts and stops and disappointments—no matter how many there were. Set your goal right now for a brand-new body and spirit. Not just "less overweight" but sleek, lean, healthy and happy. You now have the map you needed to reach your destination in record time and to maintain your results.

Not everyone will get to experience the excitement of driving a Ferrari, Lamborghini or other exotic vehicle…but YOU can really feel a similar thrill, because nothing compares to the exhilaration a TurboCharged body will deliver. See it, feel it, go for it and don't stop from this day forward until you get all the way to your finish line and trophy!

If you continue to follow the eight steps, as described in this book, you will continue to improve even though you may be eating unlimited amounts of TurboCharged foods. We know that may sound unbelievable, yet it is true. Your metabolism will have been converted to easily rely on fat for energy and to burn it from internal or external sources quickly and efficiently along with the natural carbohydrates from fruits and vegetables. Today Dian, at 5'6" tall, requires 2,475 calories to maintain her 117-119 pound body at 13.5-13.9% body fat. This is 700 calories more than the standard formula, which is 15 calories for every pound of body weight to maintain! If at any time you notice some unwanted fat showing up (a rise of 1% or greater), go back to the basics. Stick with TurboCharging foods and work the steps. Read this book again! This is the reason we have asked you to keep it for yourself. It will always be a valuable reference and contains all the information you need to keep your incredible new body and health for as long as you live. Refer to it often.

These eight simple steps will stand the test of time because they work *with* your body and not *against* it. Our bodies have the exact same needs today that have allowed the human race to exist for hundreds of thousands of years. This program, collectively, addresses those needs. And that, my friend, sums up the beauty of TurboCharged.

Questions & Answers

We have finished outlining each of the Steps that will get you to your absolute most healthy and shapely body possible: A physique that is easy to maintain for the rest of your life. That said, there might be a few questions lingering in the back of your mind. Let's try to address them.

Why didn't you include sample menus or meal plans like every other diet book?

TurboCharged is not like any other diet program. It is principle based and extremely simple. Because of this, perfect meals are also extremely simple. Ideally you eat only one type of food at a time (or meal). No recipes are required. Even with a 90/10% meal, there's not much thought or planning required other than your choice within the TurboCharged foods. TurboCharged is based on a diet of natural proteins, fruits and vegetables. If you stick with these foods and avoid complicated combining (traditional recipes) it is most effective and easy to incorporate. If you carefully read the book, you will find it does contain many suggestions for variety. However, you must remember our bodies and digestive systems evolved over hundreds of thousands of years with this very way of eating and these foods only. Eating the TurboCharged way will revive your taste buds and you will learn to enjoy and relish these natural and healthy foods and the "meals" you create with them. Your energy level will dramatically increase and will remain stable along with your sense of well-being. You will now be eating to live and no longer living to eat.

Is TurboCharged really healthy?

What exactly is a healthy diet? We can only define this as a diet that keeps us at optimal body composition and efficiency. Tell your doctor you want all your essential biomarkers tested. Get a complete check-up prior to beginning TurboCharged. Then follow the program in earnest for 10 to 30 days. See how you feel. Get another check-up and new blood tests done. The comparison will give you all the proof you need to know that TurboCharging is the ultimate, simple and easy way to improve both your physique and health.

Is the TurboCharged program OK for my children?

Yes, absolutely! The more TurboCharged foods and snacks they eat, the healthier they will be. This is actually the best thing you can do for your kids. Remember, you don't want to force-feed them. When children are really hungry they will let you know and when they do, you should provide them with the kind of foods that will TurboCharge them, keep them healthy and at an ideal weight and body composition. Get them drinking water, not juice. Purge your home of all the junk food responsible for our growing number of fat children. Children or even teenagers should not use the lower-calorie, SuperHighway approach. Let them eat as much as they want, filling up with TurboCharged foods and snacks along with the other guidelines. Nature and the innate intelligence of their bodies will take care of the rest. Fresh fruits, vegetables, eggs, cheese and fattier meats and fish will help growing children remain strong and healthy. Scrambled eggs in low-carb wraps, simple omelets or frit-tatas, along with fattier plant foods like nuts and avocados (think whole, sliced or chopped up in guacamole) are tasty and just what their active lifestyles require. Helping children develop an awareness of healthy and unhealthy food is important. When speaking with kids, don't focus on body fat. Instead, focus on eating foods that build strong healthy bodies, explaining that junk foods will zap strength and health and ultimately add fat. Hand them a box of raisins, an organic cheese stick, dates with peanut butter stuffed inside and a frozen or ripe banana—then tell them to get outside and PLAY!

We like to have dinner as a family. It seems like this evening meal is the only time we can all sit down together for some quality time. Can I still do TurboCharged?

Congratulations! Gathering daily for a family dinner is a long-standing tradition in many cultures and it really is a good one. These days, with our busy schedules, we seem to be losing this precious and rewarding time. Continue your family dinners! You are setting a great example for your children and others. Yes, the whole family can become TurboCharged. Gradually start preparing dinners using the TurboCharged foods and nutrient separation guidelines. Roast a chicken or broil a steak and serve with vegetables. Make a hearty bean and vegetable soup. Be sure to have plenty of grapes or other easy-to-eat fruit handy along with plenty of water. We think your family will really begin to enjoy eating like this and you will all be much healthier. In addition, the SuperHighway or Expressway versions of TurboCharged are so flexible, as is Cruise Control, adults will be able to follow it and still enjoy TurboCharged family dinners. If you need to lose some body fat, just eat very little during the day (100-calorie suggestions) and follow all the other steps. At dinnertime, if the meal is TurboCharged, feel free to sit down, eat as much as you need and really enjoy it! You will be setting the perfect example for your family!

After I become TurboCharged, does my body always use fat for energy?

As we have discussed, prior to TurboCharging, most people derive the majority of their energy from a constant supply of sugar provided in various forms by their diet. Because of this and the chronically elevated insulin levels it creates, the transition or "switch" to using body fat will not work the way nature intended it. A diet containing sugar, refined carbohydrates and grains can shut the process down totally. The steps in TurboCharged retrain your body to easily source your body fat (and fat from your diet) along with the natural sugars ingested from the fruits and vegetables we are now eating for your energy needs. You develop a true hybrid system, which will automatically and easily use all sources of available energy either from diet or body fat in a seamless fashion. When you follow the steps during periods when you eat less, instead of converting lean body mass for energy, you will easily access your own body fat. This will be obvious from the resulting lack of hunger and elevated feelings of well-being.

Is there a minimum amount of protein that should be consumed per day?

Protein is important not just for tissue repair and replacement but also for proper operation of the immune system. This said, we could go fairly long without "complete" protein (chicken, fish, beef, tofu or cheese) in the diet. However, in the ultimate absence of an adequate amount of complete dietary protein, the body will eventually turn to lean body mass for its supply. TurboChargers avoid this by getting at least 20-25 grams daily or more than this once every 3-4 days. If you are a high-level or professional athlete who is already TurboCharged and you exercise strenuously on a daily basis, you may need 100 grams or more per day (which is a topic for another book). Protein deficiency in the West is extremely rare and not something you should be concerned about. In fact, eating protein beyond your actual body requirement will slow the rate of fat loss. Eating protein in excess of your actual daily caloric requirement will stop fat loss. When Turbochargers reach their optimal body composition they can begin eating more natural dietary fats found in whole proteins, nuts, seeds, avocados and olives. A Turbocharged body will readily use these fats for energy requirements along with the natural carbohydrates found in the fruits and vegetables.

What do I say if someone says that TurboCharged is just another high-protein/low-carbohydrate diet or that very low-calorie diets will make me fat?

This is simple. You say, "You obviously have not read the book! I have no time to speak with you about my success if you don't choose to buy the book and spend two hours to read it. Once you have, I'd love to have an informed discussion with you." Life is filled with naysayers and people who have failed so many times on traditional "weight loss" programs and have accepted defeat. We find they often like company. Spouses, friends, children, co-workers and strangers can all, whether intentionally or not, do their best to try to get you to quit. Whether their comments are based on ignorance or doubt or feeling threatened or competitive, their noise is irrelevant to you. Don't listen. Stay the course. You don't have to be accommodating. Simply remember to tell them: "Read the book." Keep your thinking like Michelangelo's. He didn't see a block of marble. He saw

David and merely chipped away the excess. Visualize your exciting new body the same way!

Isn't obesity genetic?

Obesity is not genetic. The primary reason your body is not functioning properly at optimal sleek and lean capacity is the result of environmental factors and unhealthy patterns of choices within family lines, along with improper diet and activity choices. These factors have caused obesity to reach epidemic proportions in Western populations. Common modern diet and exercise advice is responsible for excess insulin release and the loss of lean muscle mass. These two factors are the primary causes of obesity today. Every diet other than TurboCharged has an inherent problem because their recommendations cause their struggling followers to store more fat while they lose lean muscle mass. The conversion of lean tissue for energy is endemic in the West and this continuous loss of lean body mass lowers basal metabolism and makes normal eating, when resumed, fattening. The common prescription for reducing excess weight is a lower-calorie diet and aerobic exercise, yet this regimen generally causes more lean-tissue loss. Aerobic exercise easily turns toward muscle for energy. This destabilizes powerful brain functions and results in extreme hunger and negative moods that trigger overeating and start a vicious cycle. Few people are aware that lack of activity, stress, dehydration, many types of exercise, lack of protein, some prescription drugs and dieting can cause the rapid breakdown of muscle to generate energy. If you TurboCharge as directed in this book, you will be losing your excess body fat and increasing your lean muscle mass ever so slightly every day, which supports your fat-loss goals and keeps you feeling happy.

Isn't TurboCharged just another glycemic index (GI) diet?

Managing insulin response is just one piece of the TurboCharged program. GI diets do not work for achieving leanness. They do seem to work better as far as improving overall health when compared to other diets. The peanut is often cited as the lowest glycemic food but a diet rich in peanuts will bring increases in body fat. The glycemic index and diets based on it look at the body's reaction to individual foods. This is helpful only if you eat one thing at a time. Eating meals containing a combination of different foods makes this information virtually useless. Fat added to any meal will reduce the insulin impact. However, the combination of fat and carbohydrate, which almost never exists in nature and is not seen in any animal diet, leads to rapid fat storage. This is an important piece of information. Large meals and particularly fat/carbohydrate meals (think French fries and burgers with buns, for example), so common today, send signals to your brain that there is an abundance of food. The response is to rapidly store body fat in preparation for future famine. TurboChargers ignore GI index (and eat lots of bananas!) and make vegetables and fruits the bulk of a meal or create a meal around a protein like fish, meat, eggs, tofu or cheese. Ideally, we keep these two food nutrient groups distinct and separate.

Won't I get the same results just giving up all carbohydrate foods and eating Atkins-style?

The short answer is definitely not! With all their bacon, burgers, butter and cheese, how many Atkins devotees do you see walking around with bodies you'd choose for your ultimate transportation vehicle? Atkins folks highly limit fruit. They think if you just avoid all carbohydrates and stuff yourself with fat and protein the problem is solved. Wrong!

You can get fat by overeating anything except fresh raw fruits and vegetables. Your body just has to work a little harder to do it when you overconsume fats and/or protein. With any extended high-protein diet, you will lose water weight and muscle mass, while you may not even lose much fat; plus you will constantly be dehydrated. Most people can't stick with strictly high-protein/fat diets due to their natural desire for something sweet. How could any diet be truly healthy that eliminates or largely curtails naturally delicious fruits that are loaded with essential nutrients and water that is perfectly efficient at transporting the nutrition to your every cell? There is no free lunch, other than your own body fat! The TurboCharged program is the simplest, easiest, fastest, most pleasurable road to a healthy lean body.

P.S.: Even the modified Atkins plans that are currently touted are wrong. They allow the gradual introduction of refined carbohydrates and this will simply lead to increasing excess insulin and ultimately fat storage.

When we restrict our calories to less than 800 per day, does the percentage of protein, carbohydrate and fat in the daily diet make any difference?

Fruits and vegetables can be eaten exclusively and you'll get plenty of nutrition. Interestingly, the human body is constantly recycling dead cells as a protein source. So if stress is minimal, very little additional protein intake is necessary (i.e., 25g/day every day or less for 1-3 days). If there is regular stress on the home or work fronts or if aerobic activity or heavy and extended weight training is being done while calories are being reduced, there can be a destabilization of hormones, and severe hunger will occur along with the need for more protein. If you are following the TurboCharged program, stress is minimized and the natural sources of protein, carbohydrates and fats tend to end up at ideal levels without much thought. Follow your instincts (and moods) and you will do fine. We've given you the guidelines—the choices are up to you.

What foods will get me TurboCharged more rapidly? Is eating mostly protein, or fat and protein, more effective than mostly fruits and vegetables?

TurboCharging seems to happen most quickly when people use fruits and vegetables with very little protein for 1-3 days followed by one or two mostly protein days. Focusing on eating fruits and vegetables seems to direct the brain to aggressively source body fat. The food proportions are less important than activity. If you are up and moving on your feet 1-3 hours per day and using very light weights 3-5 times during the day as well, the body will turn to fat stores for energy immediately and thus requires very little protein or other food. The protein used will be replenished when extra protein is supplied. You will know your body is relying on fat stores when you feel good and have lots of energy. This can only be accomplished by including walking and the one-minute weight routines used during waking hours. All things being equal, whatever makes one feel the best with the least hunger is the best for fat burning.

Considering whole foods are generally best, which would you consider best for fat burning:
- **160 calories of whey protein and fruit drink (high protein, low fat, some carbohydrate)**
- **160 calories consisting of 2 whole eggs (more fat than protein)**
- **160 calories of sardines or some other fish (more protein than fat)**
- **160 calories of steamed broccoli (low protein, low fat, complex carbohydrate)**

All of the above will work well, but everyone seems to require different nutrients, so variety is best. We do not need all nutrients every day, as our bodies work much like a bank: depositing extra nutrients for future use, lending them out when they are needed, and waiting for repayment in the form of a nutritious meal. Rotating fruits, legumes, veggies, meats, eggs and cheese will provide complete nutrition. Don't rule out steak or other beef products, because eating them once or twice a week might make a big positive difference for you on multiple levels including supplying B vitamins, chiefly B12. A favorite aspect of the TurboCharged program is that there are so many different ways to reach a personal destination.

People often say, "I find that the excessive fluid intake makes me feel and look bloated." Can you comment on that?

Dehydration is often a very misleading signal that body fat is being lost when it is not. This is why TurboChargers record their results by measuring body fat, which is the only part of your body you want to reduce. Beginner TurboChargers sometimes think because they ate this or that, they woke up "thinner" because of it. In actuality, they woke up *looking* thinner because the foods are absorbing so much fluid from essential tissues that have now been drained of water to aid digestion. They look thinner because they are extremely dehydrated. This is rarely discussed or recognized in diet literature and the consequence is that goals of health, fabulosity and leanness are promptly sabotaged by this mirage. Some novice TurboChargers say: "I did this intensive aerobic session and was leaner afterward." No, this is not accurate. Dehydration resulted, making the person look thinner (yet not healthier). After either the next meal or fluid intake, the body will appear the same (or worse) than before. After following the TurboCharged program for a short period, your body will be operating properly. Any experience of bloating will vanish and maximum fluid intake will no longer be necessary.

I heard that drinking too much water could kill you! Is that true?

If you drink a gallon of water within a half hour, as some highly publicized runners once did, you could die. However, we urge TurboChargers to drink up to a quart of water about four times a day, and this is not lethal. Training programs for every branch of our military advocate increased water consumption prior to any stressful activity. The average day in our modern lifestyle is loaded with stress, so fill up your tank and get TurboCharged. We often hear that too much water is dangerous for those who have high blood pressure. Technically speaking, anything and everything that people with high blood pressure are currently doing and eating is dangerous! High blood pressure is a ticking time bomb. So what's really crazy? Drinking some water or continuing to indulge in the very habits that are wreaking havoc with your health? You do not have to guzzle a quart in five minutes! You can enjoy it over a period of an hour, with your minute routines and TurboCharged meals. Your blood pressure will drop to ideal levels. It naturally drops very quickly if you go as long as possible using only body fat instead of eating at regular meal times when you don't need to. Nothing is worse for high blood pressure than grains, large meals and meal combos. Many beginner TurboChargers are pleasantly surprised with the quick drop in blood pressure that results from eating correctly and being better hydrated, as this program endorses.

Note: If you are currently taking medication for high blood pressure and get light-headed after starting TurboCharged, contact your physician because you may need to reduce or stop taking your medication as your blood pressure normalizes.

You are telling us "don't follow the food pyramid" that is based on grains and breads and is endorsed by the American Medical Association, the U.S. Government and the American Heart Association. Are you two crazy?

Well, this is a very good question. We have not been mentally assessed! We'd like to flip the table with a quote from Hugh Tunstall-Pedoe, the spokesperson for one of the largest cardiovascular studies ever undertaken. "If you do a study…you rush off and publish it. If you don't, unless you have great confidence in yourself, you worry that perhaps you didn't measure something properly, or perhaps you'd better keep quiet, or perhaps there's something you haven't thought about. And, by doing this, there is a risk of myths becoming self-perpetuating. There are people who want to believe that if we find anything less than 100% correlation between traditional risk factors (and trends in heart disease), we are somehow traitors to the cause of public health, and what we say should be suppressed, and we should be ashamed of ourselves. Whereas we are asking a perfectly reasonable question and what we came up with were results. That is what science is all about."

We believe in studying science, reading research and assessing facts. We have had the opportunity to speak with literally hundreds of scientifically minded people during our collective 30 years+ working with innovative, cutting-edge biotechnology, specialty/pharmaceutical and medical device companies. TurboCharged is supported by books along with thousands of research papers on nutrition, health, anthropology, stress, food combining, nutrient separation, fasting, VLCDs, physical fitness/exercise and countless other topics by some of the world's foremost scientific researchers in the areas of obesity, cardiovascular disease, diabetes and longevity. (See Supplemental Reading List on page 187 and research articles posted at www.turbocharged.us.com.) From reading and assessing a tremendous amount of others' research and work, we believe our conclusions regarding activity and food choices while reducing body fat are well-supported and highly substantiated. We believe and live what we are sharing with you, our treasured reader. If we have improved just one life, prevented one heart attack, helped someone find love that they thought was elusive because of their excess fat, improved someone's body image, helped someone get off a lifetime of prescription drugs or any of the other wonderful things we know can result from people getting TurboCharged, the years we have spent collaborating that culminated in this book have been very worthwhile. We know in our hearts that the truth speaks loudly and proudly. We know that if you get through your first 10 days of TurboCharged, you will be well on your way to celebrating your remaining years on Earth in a fabulous body with the ultimate benefit of greatly improved health. You will be inspired to reach your goal. Your constant hunger will have disappeared and you will be feeling simply fantastic. You can do it. And when you do, others will ask, "How did you get such an awesome body?" You will tell them, "You'll have to buy and read *TurboCharged.*"

I'm only 25. Will it really work for me too?

The science behind TurboCharged is solid and the eight steps will work for everyone regardless of their age or anything else! We all have the same DNA and anthropological heritage, and if you go back far enough, we come from the same family tree! Just get started and prove it to yourself. You will be amazed too!

My trainer says this program is all wrong...

If some aerobic or fitness trainer starts giving you nutritional advice, or, frankly, anyone else who spends hours a day exercising, day after day, stop listening (or just push the ejector seat button ☺). Most likely, their "experience" is going to refer you to the usual mantra: Don't go below 1,600 calories a day, eat balanced meals, be sure to have plenty of grains, snack bars count as great meal replacements, and exercise 60-90 minutes daily. Those suggestions don't work, unless you prefer to feel hungry and cranky all the time. Only about 5% of us are able to keep up vigorous exercise routines while limiting or reducing calories. The other 95% of us fail. Yet all diet and fitness gurus keep pushing out the same formula in their diet books with a few new twists on old themes. For most of us, this formula just doesn't work. Once you are on the road to TurboCharging, you will find you will adapt easily and quickly as your tastes for the wrong foods go away and your body's natural desires return with a vengeance. Your strong, energetic, lean body coupled with ideal blood pressure, low triglycerides, rising HDL and other improvements can all be documented with a full blood panel and will provide you with all the proof anyone needs. Every day when you get up, take a look at yourself in the mirror. The reflection will prove how well you have taken control of your body, health and life.

No aerobics and I'll lose fat? Are you sure?

It has been reported in numerous studies that dieters who use aerobics (50% VO2 max) can experience a lower base metabolic rate (BMR) (about 10%), and almost 50% of total weight loss can be lean muscle mass when combined with a 40% calorie-restricted diet, even with moderate-to-high protein intake. Whether or not you understand that bit of science is irrelevant. Just know—it is not good. What is more significant about this "aerobics to lose weight phenomenon" is how common this strategy is used in Western populations for weight loss. We believe this is a significant reason why most who exercise vigorously and reduce calories still fail in their efforts to reduce body fat. Virtually every major medical and dietetic association is giving out bad prescriptions when they recommend the above regimen of aerobic exercise and reduced caloric intake. This combo results in loss of lean muscular tissue, which means you are losing weight but getting flabbier or just "shrinking"! Granted, there is no doubt that proper nutrition combined with aerobic and anaerobic exercise can contribute substantially to overall fitness and health, but to get TurboCharged, these activities are simply not appropriate while you are cutting calories if you want long-term success. We repeat: Get TurboCharged first. Then do the marathons, triathlons, or whatever else you want to do. Your ultimate performance will be better for it.

Can I jog instead of walk? Or even better, start marathon training since I feel so good?

Get TurboCharged first, which will convert your engines to easily run on fat for energy instead of unnecessary sugar or, worse, your lean body mass. Jogging, running or any other form of aerobic exercise will simply make you want to eat more. Even if you run just a short time, your appetite goes through the roof and you will experience constant hunger. The same is true for any type of stressful activity. Eroding lean mass as a result of physical or mental stress causes an assault on the brain's protective mechanisms. The brain's answer to almost any stress is hunger. Consequently, the brain triggers every appetite mechanism at its disposal because until about 3,000 years ago all of the stresses experienced were related to certain death. Starvation, survival and sudden exertion often meant being chased by an animal or engaging in hand-to-hand lethal combat! We cannot fight these mechanisms with aerobic exercise and ever succeed. TurboCharged provides the highest levels of nutrition along with the only activities you will ever need to reach a sleek, lean, attractively muscular body. If you really desire to run a marathon, please start training only after you are lean. (Notice a theme here?)

But I thought fat burning increased significantly after aerobic exercise?

Aerobics cannot be fueled sufficiently by body fat because the conversion time of body fat to the instant fuel required to maintain aerobic or anaerobic-induced stress is longer. For the first 20 minutes give or take, blood sugar is the fuel and then lean mass is converted into sugar. At a certain point the mix becomes about 50/50 body fat and lean mass. Being stationary requires blood sugar only and rarely body fat. Studies show that for hours after aerobics, body fat becomes a primary fuel and many advocates point to this. However, most people eat or drink sugary "energy replacements" after exercising and this negates any potential extra fat burning and at the same time sets the stage for insatiable hunger that can last for hours and perhaps days if the cycle keeps repeating. The goal of TurboCharging is to reach the metabolic zone that sources body fat as the primary fuel. You could compare it to the theme of Goldilocks and the Three Bears: Standing or sitting will not release body fat—it is not enough. Aerobic activity requires more sugar than being sedentary—but this is too much. Walking, however, is a superior fat-burning activity and is just right. Walking allows body fat to easily convert to fuel as long as you have been drinking enough water, as we recommend. In all scenarios, stressing all muscle groups with walking and the one-minute weight-bearing exercises will prevent lean-mass loss and promote the continual use of body fat for fuel. If you insist on doing aerobic activity, get lean first! Otherwise, you will simply become another "fit-fat person," meaning you may be able to do superior physical feats—but you'll be carrying more body fat than is healthy and you will not be lean. All self-proclaimed athletes that work this program claim that they got leaner and their respective performance improved.

From the female perspective, what is the most important thing I can do for success?

First off, accept the natural shape of your body. Whether you are small-boned, built like an Amazonian woman, tall like a Somalian model, short, average, whatever, you can look absolutely fabulous once TurboCharged and you will be much healthier. Whatever body parts are naturally big or small on you, work them to your advantage. Be grateful you've got a body that you can shape. Next, focus on fat. You may TurboCharge and still have larger legs because you've got wonderful muscles propelling you forward. How fabulous! Maybe your legs are like sticks. TurboCharging will make them fit and shapely sticks. Women come in all shapes and sizes. We love every form we've ever seen. Our focus is eliminating all your unnecessary body fat, which causes all sorts of problems. The biggest challenge most women face as they age is always a lower-body issue. Women in jobs requiring them to sit all day have lost 10-30 pounds of muscle from their legs and buttocks. These are the muscles responsible for most of our metabolism. Women need to focus on walking and doing squats and lunges for their minute workouts to get these muscles back. Fitness trainers who have women working their arms until they are very defined are misleading them. This may look nice in a little black dress, but these muscles have minimal impact on fat-burning metabolism. TurboChargers focus on strengthening all their muscles, which will greatly accelerate the speed of fat burning. Women who concentrate on their upper bodies are wasting their time since legs and rear ends have greater amounts of lean muscle tissue. For women, the lower-body is the key to regaining a youthful metabolism and much lower body fat. What women need most is some type of weighted backpack combined with more walking. This will return the lean tissue to the lower body. Patience is required because these lower body parts have declined from years of minimal use. TurboCharged routines involving lower body strengthening and especially walking are key to boosting metabolism, not to mention that strong legs and tushies greatly increase energy, strength and mood while looking great too!

Why do some women look really cut?

Women who get their body-fat percentage below 12% (usually from excess aerobic exercise) begin to look freakish and will gain a lot of weight when they burn out or have an injury, accident or too much anxiety. Then hunger returns with a roar. Women should not try to become as lean as a man. Doing so will have a negative impact on their hormones. A 13.5-18% body-fat level is ideal and healthy. In this range, enough fat has been eliminated to insure a long life and good health as well as vigor, pride, sex appeal and ease of maintenance. Over time, without trying, if you continue eating plenty of TurboCharged foods, while following all the steps, you will continue to cut up and get leaner—while eating more calories! Don't be surprised if, like many others, you start to believe that TurboCharging has accessed the Fountain of Youth. On an average of 2,300 calories or more a day coupled with walking and 3-5 mini-workouts daily, Dian's body has dropped this past year from 18% to 13.7% body fat according to her Tanita scale. Again, this has happened while eating Cruise Control foods including cheese, but not crackers, and drinking red wine. Get to lean, shift into Cruise Control and stick with the steps. You will be amazed by how your body continues to shape itself—often reversing years of neglect.

I'm an athlete. What do I do since aerobics are a large part of my training?

If you are reading this book, chances are your current regimen has still left you with stubborn body fat. Maybe you are a "fit-fat person" or perhaps you're just looking for that extra edge. If you are not as lean as you would like to be, some changes to your routine are in order. It is really helpful to get TurboCharged before participating in any high-stress activities. Consider reducing your training in the off-season to concentrate on getting lean. All stressful exercise is counterproductive to getting lean. Try backing off the intensity when your schedule allows. That said, if you must continue your training, the best way to minimize the stress created by aerobic exercise is to eat a lot of TurboCharged foods. Stay away from those sugary sports drinks and other "replenishing foods" and you will not only start getting leaner but also, as an added benefit, your performance will reach new heights.

Can I ever eat a bag of chips or a bowl of ice cream again?

Ice cream, chips, a warm piece of bread just out of the oven or a piece of cake, whatever your preference—yes, if you want, you can eat it again. The goal is to wait until you are TurboCharged. Once you have gotten to the healthy fat-burning physique you want, if the urge strikes, or your mind tricks you into believing that an event would be more special with a sweet treat, indulge. But you might be surprised. Many TurboChargers report that the "special treat" has somehow lost some of its specialness. Sugary sweets actually do become less desirable and a combo of sugar and fat can leave an unpleasant taste on the tongue. Once you have reached your goal, you, like most people living the TurboCharged lifestyle, may find that your new eating plan and activity routine is quite enjoyable and you feel great physically and mentally. It will become something you "don't want to mess with." If you do the program according to the outline of this book, you will notice there is virtually no hunger, even from day one. By day four or five, your willpower becomes incredible and your desire for "outlawed" foods simply vanishes. If you contrast these feelings to those felt when not on the plan, your weight was up and your mood was down. You may just realize the best "reward" is your new physique along with great spirits and not that sugary treat that anyone (including you!) can easily have. You now truly eat to live, not live to eat.

Does popcorn count as a vegetable?

Popcorn is not a TurboCharged vegetable! Popcorn is usually a high sugar/fat combination, especially the movie-theatre variety (which FYI has no redeeming "food" value whatsoever!) As such, it is a serious detour, guaranteed to spike your insulin levels and leave you feeling hungrier. Instead, you might like to try some pumpkin seeds including the shells. Pumpkin seeds are about 120 calories per quarter-cup serving. You really need to eat one at a time since it takes lots of time to fully chew them well before swallowing. These are really delicious and a very satisfying snack. As most brands are salted this will cause some fluid retention (which is NOT the same as hydration!). Make sure you are still drinking plenty of water or some other non-caloric, healthy liquid. Why pumpkin seeds when nuts and seeds aren't listed as TurboCharged foods while reducing? The difference with pumpkin seeds is that you eat the shells, so most of the meal is fiber. P.S.: If you have children, get them to try their own pack of pumpkin seeds. You will be pleasantly surprised as most are fascinated with "eating shells" and enjoy this tasty TurboCharged snack.

Do I have to count M&Ms, Hershey's Kisses or Tic Tacs if I eat them? They are so small.

One novice TurboCharger gave us a good chuckle. He emailed us, wondering why he had stalled. He swore he was sticking with the plan. So we asked him to give us a list of what he was eating. Sure enough, the list as written was TurboCharged food all the way. After a few more conversations and emails, he slipped. Quite casually he asked: "M&Ms couldn't hurt me, could they?" Well, problem found! YES, something as tiny as a few M&Ms can ruin your progress. M&Ms, Skittles, SweeTarts, Tic Tacs, jellybeans, chocolate covered nuts or pretzels and Swedish Fish (along with everything else that you know to be candy!) are essentially pure sugar and they will shut down your TurboCharger. Even worse, because they are pure sugar, they will not even begin to make you feel satiated. You would have to eat an awful lot to feel full. Candy is the worst form of a simple carbohydrate, along with processed breads, cereals and other grains. These carbohydrates are digested very rapidly and will raise your blood sugar quickly. Then your blood sugar will drop just as quickly, leaving you craving more. Subsequently you just keep shoveling them in. FYI: To be absolutely clear, Peanut M&Ms don't count as nuts either!

Are artificial sweeteners allowed?

We are not big advocates of artificial sweeteners. However, after the brain and cells have become so adjusted to insulin "jolts" produced by a traditional diet, it is very difficult for some to be satisfied after a meal without something "sweet," even if just artificially so. Due to past conditioning, some of us feel intense urges for sweets. TurboChargers can initially become road-blocked when we say anything negative about diet drinks or coffee with artificial sweeteners, so we pulled back on our criticism. As you have probably read, the research is very much still out on whether artificially sweetened foods and drinks help or hinder body-fat loss, along with whether or not they cause health problems. Nonetheless, people still seem to want them and rage against all warnings about artificial sweets as a replacement for real sweets. Chocolates or other candies that are artificially sweetened are not a great solution. Any amount of fresh, raw fruit is better, but we have conceded on this issue because it doesn't seem to do much damage and definitely promotes lower insulin than a sugar-laden dessert or candy. If you must, we recommend a small amount of dark chocolate, maybe with some almonds, sweetened with malitol. At least this way you can also pick up a few extra antioxidants!

I've been sticking with the TurboCharged steps, but last night I ate some bread, sugar or any other refined carbohydrate and I think I look more "defined" today. Is this possible?

This is an interesting subject and may be one of the more important issues related to the growing incidence of body fat, obesity and disease. We have had many conversations with people who say, "I had such and such for dinner and the next day I could see a definite difference in my body that showed I had lost weight." We have to explain that they woke up more dehydrated than usual because sugary carbohydrates, and especially fat/carbohydrate combination foods, are highly dehydrating! The same phenomenon occurs when beginning TurboChargers insist on their aerobic workouts. They claim they can see a large difference later and that this means they have lost body fat. "No," we must explain, they are dehydrated and may also have lost muscle. Conversely, due to the amount of water we recommend that you consume, some complain that they are bloated. Well, listen up! Having a full tank of water is very good for you. Water aids immensely in filling up your stomach. This is essential for TurboChargers because your stomach is most likely almost double the size that Nature intended due to years of overeating. An unfilled stomach will not release satiety hormones, signaling the brain that enough food has been consumed. Remember too that fat cells are light, composed of only 25-31% water, but muscle cells are heavier with 70-75% water. So fill your tank with 16 to 32 ounces of water, stick with lean proteins of any kind, along with fresh fruits and vegetables, and become TurboCharged.

Can I ever eat a fast-food burger again?

The short answer is yes. Have that ¼ or ½-pound burger and skip the bun and dressing while stacking up on the tomatoes, pickles and onions. If you crave the cheese, go ahead and enjoy it without the bun or sugary ketchup. Just remember, French fries do not count as vegetables! Stay away from fast-food joints until your willpower is such that you can pass on the bun, fries and regular sodas!

Can I reward myself?

Yes, but how about redefining "rewards"? Rather than indulging in a huge piece of chocolate cake topped with ice cream and whipped cream, seek out some non-food prizes that reward and inspire you. Something as simple as closing your eyes and visualizing yourself in a skimpy bathing suit on the beach might work. Call a friend and set a date to converse and relax. Book a massage or facial. If you need a physical reward, buy a great book, go load up your iPod or MP3 player with some rocking music or buy a sexy shirt in the size you intend to achieve. Find something that inspires you and go for it! Non-food rewards are really more rewarding. The best reward is a healthy, fit, sleek, lean, awe-inspiring body for the rest of your life. A body that looks great in whatever clothes you decide to wear. A body that has glowing skin. A body that is energized.

What substitutions can I make?

TurboChargers make no substitutions. Substitutions are not part of the plan. Fruits, vegetables, fish, meats, beans, some nuts and cheese, two tablespoons of half-and-half in coffee or tea, a scoop or two of pure protein powder, lots of water and other no-calorie beverages are it. If you are confused, follow this simple rule: If it comes in a package not designed by Mother Nature, it is best to skip it, especially during your fat-loss TurboCharged phase. NOTE: We make an exception for protein powder because it helps provide essential protein for those on the SuperHighway plan. Protein powder should only be considered as a "tool" during this phase—not a permanent substitute for real foods as offered by Nature. Half-and-half is our other "packaged" exception. We believe up to two tablespoons in a cup of coffee, no more than twice a day, may provide the fat and satisfaction some of us desire—without triggering insulin spikes.

How about all those special "diet" foods, teas, supplements, potions and pills that get touted on TV and magazine covers?

TurboChargers are wise. We do not believe the hype that any food or substance is a "wonder food" or "magic potion." We believe in a variety of natural foods, full of naturally occurring water and nutrients for building health and maintaining a sleek, lean physique. TurboChargers avoid supplements and other fads. If you read enough literature on any supplement, you will find 50% of the articles singing its praises and 50% issuing warnings. At best, information on supplements is contradictory and distracting, and most claims may be disproved or disputed in later studies. We believe supplements, more often than not, are a waste of your money. If you really insist, find a good multivitamin and take one a day.

What about prepared foods?

If you need another reason why whole, fresh foods such as fruits, vegetables, fish and lean meats, prepared at home, are best for you…here you go: MSG. Studies show there is a link between the flavor enhancer monosodium glutamate (MSG) and weight gain. The additive seems to interfere with your body's ability to regulate your appetite. Chinese restaurants aren't the only places you will find MSG. Unfortunately, it is a common ingredient in many canned foods, soups, and salad dressings and even smoked almonds. Scan nutrition labels and know that manufacturers realize consumers are wising up to the detrimental effects of MSG, so they use other names to confuse us. Watch not only for monosodium glutamate but also hydrolyzed soy protein and autolyzed yeast. And get this—even "vegetable broth" is a new label for MSG to sneak into your body.

Have any easy suggestions for dining out?

No TurboCharged man or woman will likely live by home cooking alone. Restaurant dining will be part of your life. The good news is, the TurboCharged program works quite well with restaurant dining. Simply turn on your computer prior to heading out to dine. Many restaurants now post their menus online. Take a moment to plan your meal according to the TurboCharged guidelines before leaving your house. This will allow more time for conversation, optimal food choices and less chance of turning off your new TurboCharged status. It also helps to fill your tank with water before getting to the restaurant so all those great smells don't distract you, causing a crash! Remember, you are a paying customer, so don't be afraid to make special requests and ask for substitutions as needed. Any good restaurant will be glad to oblige. Finally, skip the bread basket or ask for it to be placed on the opposite end of the table.

My mate works outdoors and I pack the breakfast and lunches for the day. It's a challenge because he (she) can't bring any food along that won't "survive" in extreme heat or cold. Everything must be packed to go. What do you recommend?

Hard-boiled eggs shouldn't be too much trouble if you peel them before packing. Eggs are higher in fat and it is best to stick with fertile, organic or omega-3 type rather than regular eggs. Fruit would work great all by itself and he can continue to eat until he is full. A thermos with a pre-mixed smoothie that includes a scoop of protein powder is another option. Turkey rolled in lettuce or cheese makes a tasty meal. Pack a salad with chopped chicken breast or some other protein with no sugar dressing. Lemon juice or vinegar with some spices with maybe a little olive oil tastes great. A bean salad with no added fat is easy. Any bean combo works well. Be creative with spices. Just a chicken breast or some leftover turkey with seasoning will create variety. Cut up celery or cucumber sticks and include a bit of raw nut butter for dunking. Fast food: grilled chicken, salad, no bread, chips or French fries. A burger with or without cheese (throwing away the bun) will work. Encourage your mate to drink more water in place of snacks. It is very important to remember that starchy carbohydrates or sugar mixed with fat are very bad combinations. That is why packaged foods are such a problem—they always have this mix. So plan on doing your own preparing and know you are helping to create a healthy, lean body.

Any tips for managing stress and mindless eating?

Tension and stress are the most oft-cited reasons for overeating. Stress will happen. It is a standard, everyday part of life. Too bad a cookie can't really solve a problem. Prepare ahead. Always keep some TurboCharged snacks such as fresh fruit around. Better yet, go through all the steps. Make a list of things you can do when your anxiety buttons get pushed: Eat some fruit, practice your meditation or visualization exercises, phone a friend, take a walk, read a good book, watch a funny movie and maybe enjoy a half-glass of wine, all of which can be positive alternatives to cookies. Writing an overdue snail mail letter to a friend, planning an exotic beach vacation and going to the store to find a new bathing suit can work, too. Be reminded: Stressed spelled backward is Desserts.

I've been on TurboCharged for two full days but I'm feeling moody, cranky, agitated. Am I doing something wrong?

If for any reason you are not feeling great after two full days, you are not eating enough! TurboChargers eat! Make a protein shake with 25 grams of protein powder blended up with fruits, ice and water or simply make sure you are having another six or so fruits as a meal.

My body-fat scale says my fat is going down, but I don't see it happening on my body. What is going on?

Keep in mind that there is a large amount of visceral (internal) fat that almost everyone is unaware of. When we wake up and do not see our bellies looking smaller we are sometimes disappointed. We see via our scales that body fat is reduced but it is a visceral fat reduction. This is most common with those who do very well and then see they still have some belly fat (however small relative to the way they were before) and ask us what is wrong. Nothing is wrong. The brain/body uses body fat from different areas at different rates. Your body knows best. Trust it!

If I'm hungry what should I do?

Before eating, you want to:

- Drink up 16-32 ounces of water;

- Brush your teeth or rinse with mouthwash or use a minty breath strip;

- Take a walk (even 5 or 10 minutes will do) and/or do a minute's worth of weight resistance;

- Visualize your sleek, lean TurboCharged physique.

Then, if you are still hungry, by all means EAT! Simply choose to eat either a piece of meat, fish, chicken, tofu or beans OR have some vegetables or fruit. Enjoy and be present with each bite. No multitasking! Anytime you feel hunger, repeat this cycle. There will be plenty of times when you notice your hunger has disappeared. Again, this is because you were more likely THIRSTY, not hungry!

Do I really need to follow all the steps to lose my body fat?

The TurboCharged program is holistic. It works *with* your body, not *against* it. It will work if you work each step. You will not get TurboCharged without the weights (or calisthenics), however brief, several times a day. Nor does the weight work by itself bring leanness or health without the other steps of TurboCharged. You could slim down with lots of incredibly strenuous weight lifting along with vigorous aerobics and limiting calories. But the stress this adds will keep zapping your mojo, make you hungry and you will not get to TurboCharged status. PLEASE DO NOT SKIP ANY STEP or feel the urge to add more "exercise". Without doing all the steps as outlined on a regular basis, especially during the first few days and until all your excess body fat is gone, your brain will fight you and the weight you lose will be mostly muscle, not fat. Each step tells your brain to hold onto muscle. Your food intake with TurboCharged foods becomes less and less important to your success. You will get TurboCharged with insulin levels so low that calories reduce automatically to enforce and return you to a sleek physique. However, even if you were eating the excellent and nutritious foods on the TurboCharged program, you will lose muscle without walking and the minute-weight resistance routines. Consider all the TurboCharged steps your collective secret weapon.

Do I need weights?

In the beginning, dumbbells are not really necessary. Look at any Marine. You can always do squats and push-ups moving only your natural body weight. Do as many as you can for only one minute. Rest if needed but don't stop until the minute is done. Hold the top position in the push-ups when you're too tired to do another rep, rest in that position for a few seconds and do a couple more. Do this every two hours or so along with consuming 16-32 ounces of water. Bingo, three to five minutes total per day! It doesn't take much, and remember that stressing your body too much is counterproductive to fat loss. This is not commonly accepted thinking, but for the moment, just take our word for it. At least until you start seeing your own results in the very near future.

How about a sample day for fast results?

TurboChargers can lose one pound of body fat per day by following these steps: Drink 16 to 32 ounces of water first thing in the morning. Eat little or no breakfast, fruit if desired, and drink more water and/or non-caloric fluid with minimal caffeine until about 11 am–noon. Intersperse a mini-weight workout for 1-2 minutes once or twice in the morning also before noon. Enjoy vegetable salad for lunch or plenty of fresh raw fruits. Do another mini-workout with weights (or your body weight) for 1-2 minutes every two or three hours throughout the afternoon. Drink more water in quantities of 16 to 32 ounces. Eat only fruit or fruits and vegetables for the rest of the day or perhaps a small protein only dinner. Finish the day with a nice herbal tea to relax into the evening and do a mini-muscle workout before bedtime. Of course, we also recommend losing your car keys. Get walking everywhere you can. If you add an hour of walking—consecutively or broken down into 10, 15 or 20-minute walks—you will succeed much more quickly. Vegetarian TurboChargers might consider eggs or fish (if personally acceptable), tofu or a handful of nuts for that evening meal. For more ideas, go back and review the sample days provided by Dian and Tom in Step #7.

I really don't want to focus on calories. Can I still get TurboCharged?

Absolutely! We urge you to never be concerned with calories. That is the power of TurboCharged. Your body actually has an internal (genetic) meter that makes the sufficient volume obvious after a few days of eating correctly with TurboCharged foods. Soon you will find you are naturally gravitating toward a very low-calorie diet. But even if you don't, you'll lose the body fat anyway if you stick with TurboCharged food choices while separating your protein meals from vegetable and fruit meals or with the 90/10% plate. Plus you must also continue, in 2-3 hour intervals, each important step of filling your tank with water, brushing and rinsing with a minty sorbitol-sweetened toothpaste or mouthwash, carefully deciding if you are really ready to eat, taking a walk, doing a minute's worth of weight resistance and a minute of visualization focusing on your soon-to-be refined physique.

Will TurboCharging be easy?

Continuing the thoughts from our previous response, the answer is unequivocally YES! TurboCharged is remarkably easy to follow. You will experience success for what may be the first time in your life or for the first time since you were a teenager! You will find yourself in a zone with your strength and personal power growing daily. You will not feel the desire for your old foods and you will really love your brand-new appearance every morning. Isn't this exciting? Won't it make you feel happy enjoying the feeling and knowing your body is thriving? Your heart and brain are fully supporting you as you fuel your body with your excess fat. Your skin looks better, your eyes are brighter, your mood is positive, buoyant, and your future is bright. You are so very close to getting all the way to lean. It is our sincere wish for you that the past be forgotten and that you will give yourself youth again and a new lease on life. The pride you will feel for working the steps will be worth it. Everything in your life will change for the better by reaching your goal. Get TurboCharged now!

Why did you call the program TurboCharged instead of Supercharged?

We're glad you asked! The simple answer is that turbochargers are more efficient than superchargers. In mechanical engines, both rely on forced induction to increase power. A supercharger, however, uses (drains) some of the power from the engine in order to do its job just like an alternator or air conditioning compressor does. A supercharger reminds us of traditional diet and exercise advice. It may get the job done but there is an unnecessary price to pay for it. If you've gotten this far in the book, you know what we're talking about. A turbocharger, on the other hand, uses the engine's exhaust gases to power itself. This is free energy! Left untapped, it would have happily exited via the exhaust pipe and muffler on its merry way into the atmosphere. Our body fat is free energy too! We only need a way to harness it and unleash the awesome power it can provide. That is the reason we prefer to be TurboCharged.

How long can a person safely and successfully continue the TurboCharged program?

Forever!

Just one final note....

Let's all strike the words "weight loss" or "losing weight" from our vocabulary forever.

If it ain't body fat loss… it just ain't no darn good! ☺

If you continue to follow the TurboCharged steps in this book, your fat-burning "switch" will be working properly. Your new hybrid body will continue to easily source fat for fuel when available or needed, your strength will increase and your metabolism will accelerate. You will charge up your virility or femininity, run cleaner and more efficiently, and slow aging while you feel free and satisfied.

Keep reading this book. Read it over and over again. There is a lot of information and more will be remembered and absorbed each time you read it thoroughly. You now have all of the tools needed to return youth, health and vitality.

Give yourself love. When you achieve your goal for a meal, for a day, for a week, for a month, give yourself love. Compliment and congratulate yourself because you deserve it. Make yourself feel warm, fuzzy and good all over when you maintain your objectives. Keep telling yourself you can do it. When you reach a lean and healthy state, you will have accomplished something incredibly rare. It means that you can literally do anything that you set your mind to achieve. This holistic plan is not just for your body. It will rejuvenate your spirit. An elevated spirit can also be a light and inspiration for others.

"Every atom of oxygen in our lungs, carbon in our muscles, calcium in our bones and iron in our blood was created inside a star before Earth was born. We are stardust." (American Museum of Natural History, New York, NY)

Go light up the world because you are a STAR!

Our Road Trip to TurboCharged

With the exact steps we have shared in these pages, we, Tom and Dian, made the decision to get super-lean quickly. Once we arrived where we wanted to be, we hit Cruise Control to maintain our new physiques. We have attained a workable discipline, but we are by no means "perfect" (as our spouses can attest!) and don't expect you to be either.

As few roads in life are perfectly straight, here we share our personal stories with you, so you can understand what we discovered on our road trip thus far through life, what we ask of ourselves, and why we hope you will follow us down this new and exciting road.

Tom's Story

I was born on Friday the 13th, which I now consider my lucky day. I am the second of five children, and grew up in Huntington Station on Long Island, New York. I now lead a very active life, but being rather slim and small-boned (along with being slightly uncoordinated), I was never active in high school sports. Nonetheless, I possessed a healthy body and spirit with an athletic predisposition. I wasn't exactly the Charles Atlas-prototype skinny kid, who bulked up to beat up the bully who kicked sand in his face, but I began lifting weights in an attempt to put some meat on my bones to impress the girls and my buddies. Flipping through body-building magazines, I was drawn to the sculpture and detail of the physiques of the men inside. To me they looked like the ideal picture of health. As I began to see results from my lifting and diet modifications, my interest in health and fitness got stronger. It became my hobby, my passion and, some say, my obsession.

Over the years, I have read hundreds of books and thousands of articles and studies. Along with continuous weight lifting, I tried running, biking and swimming, which naturally led me to take part in triathlons. I tried almost every new diet that came along with claims of better health, performance or longevity. For example, after my father suffered a heart attack, I went on the Pritikin Diet that his doctor recommended. If it was good enough for Dave Scott, a successful U.S. triathlete who won the Ironman Triathlon in Hawaii six times between 1980 and 1987, I thought it might do wonders for me.

Somewhere along the way, my younger sister Dian and I realized we had similar interests and began collaborating and experimenting with new diet and exercise regimens. We were always reading books and comparing notes on our discoveries, revelations and disappointments. Although family and friends considered us health nuts, we never thought we were as healthy as we could be. We both looked good. However, I always wanted the bodybuilder look, yet could never build up that much muscle or get lean enough to really show off what muscle I had.

By all conventional standards, I ate right, exercised, slept well and even practiced Transcendental Meditation, yet in my mid 30s my doctor told me my cholesterol was too high. I tried *Fit for Life, Natural Hygiene, Atkins, The Zone, Body Rx, Body for Life*, etc… I even tried an all-raw vegan diet followed by an all-raw animal based diet. Regardless of the diet followed,

I never felt much different and I still had excess body fat that kept me from reaching optimal health. I was one of many fit-fat people (people who exercise a lot but don't have the body to show for it).

In 1996, my wife Janet and I each left jobs we had worked for 20 years and headed west to California. I had a new occupation in finance and a new location to explore. I continued exercising but my weight gradually crept up to 193 pounds. I didn't look fat and my Harley-riding friends told me I looked buff in my sleeveless tee shirts. The weight was spread out evenly. However, I knew I was pretty chunky. More exercise and dieting kept me yo-yoing between 175 and 185 pounds. Every September, I weighed my lowest and proceeded to gain back 10 to 12 pounds over the holidays, leading up to the New Year and another resolution to lose weight and get lean.

In 2008, I began reading more about the evolutionary concepts espoused by Dr. Loren Cordain, Mark Sisson, Mark Davis, Ray Audette, and others who each focused on "primordial" diets promoting more meat eating while limiting grain consumption. I compared these ideas to the work of raw vegan guru Gabriel Cousens, M.D. and my bodybuilding friend Charlie Abel, who wrote *The Raw Food Bodybuilding Training Manual,* both of whom eat only raw fruits, vegetables and nuts. Each of these camps take a totally different approach to how and exactly what you should eat as well as with their perspectives on exercise. In spite of their obvious differences, I was intrigued by some of the interesting similarities and what seemed to be equally good results.

Building on these "evolutionist" thinkers and the shoulders of the many who have experimented and written before us, like Herbert Shelton's "food combining" principles; Doctors Stillman, Atkins, Pescatore and all the high-protein advocates; Gary Taubes' "Good Calories, Bad Calories" concepts; Larry North's interesting mini-exercises; the basic walking principles from the American Heart Association; and hundreds of others, Dian and I began synthesizing everything from our years of study, along with plenty of trial-and-error experimentation. We spoke with every doctor, scientist or researcher who would speak with us. We like to think we have honed the knowledge we gained from reading and conversations, and taken the best concepts offered to date by anyone and everyone to create a simple program for losing excess fat very quickly with an absolute minimum of traditional exercise.

Using the eight easy Steps in this book, each day I became leaner and my strength increased. Dian and I continued experimenting and inviting our friends and family along in the process. Everyone was getting similar results, often with totally different food selections. Ultimately we were both convinced our collective program was special and knew we needed to spread the word, which is what you now have in your hands.

These days, people ask me all the time: "How did you get so lean, and how do you keep it up?" No matter how complete an answer I try to give them, it never seems to be sufficient. For one thing, in the midst of my explanation, most people think they get it, and almost always jump in with, "Oh, it's like this diet or that diet." In truth, it is not like any diet you've ever heard of or tried before. That's why we needed to write this book.

Dian's Story

Over the past 30 years, I have lived my life as a meditating vegetarian entrepreneur. I have a doctorate in nutrition, the highest certification level as a hypnotherapist and have served on the New York City chapter of the American Heart Association. I have worked, written or lectured on a broad variety of health, stress management and longevity topics and along the way have started and owned businesses in finance and marketing, health, publishing, automotive, entertainment and fashion.

I'm the fourth of the five Griesel children. Our parents followed the advice of the Surgeon General. They did not smoke, they ate less meat, and substituted margarine for butter (not something that we advise). We were quite surprised when our dad, who was always active, had his first heart attack at age 60 and ultimately died of coronary artery disease at age 78. Our mom Jane is super-slim and lives like a teenager at 81 with her husband Bernie. She has been extremely active all her life—running after five kids will help that! An early advocate of Dr. Irwin M. Stillman's ketogenic diet, whenever she needed to lose a couple of pounds she simply cut the bread out of her diet, ate lots of tuna with cottage cheese, hand-scrubbed the floors and headed to the garden. No question Tom and I were fortunate to grow up with such strong role models for moderation and self-discipline.

Starting in 1977, I managed health clubs and helped introduce the masses to both Nautilus weight workouts and racquetball. In the early 80s, I appeared in three foreign films and had a custom tee shirt design business. This all segued into a detour. I moved into Manhattan, where I began a career in the entertainment sponsorship industry.

Although it was a fun, exciting and highly "entertaining" period in my life, I have to admit that I had too many all-nighters and succumbed too often to the temptations that I also witnessed derailing many major talents. By age 24, I was a poor example of health and certainly not heading toward longevity. I decided to get back on the health track, and began my search for a healthy body and more peaceful spirit in earnest. The possibility of finding the path to ultimate health, a long life and happiness became my consummate passion. By 1987, I had begun reading everything I could find regarding stress and its effects, as well as happiness, meditation, hypnosis, and theories about the ideal ways to eat and exercise for a healthier, less-stressed and longer life.

One of my first teachers was T. C. Fry, who offered a course in Natural Hygiene. The "health" community pilloried Mr. Fry as a fraud for his teachings on health and motivation. Nonetheless, I found his coursework fascinating and read every book he wrote. Soon after I began reading everything I could find by Herbert Shelton, Arnold Ehret, and William Banting—all of whom wrote about the simple requirements for health in the 1800s. I started building my library, covering every other author, scientist, researcher, doctor and health faddist, mainstream or not, wanting to deeply understand everything there was to know about body fat, health, stress and longevity from past theories, trends and current thinking. Today, over 1,800 books line my shelves and the collection is ever-expanding.

By the mid-1990s the health, stress management and longevity articles I was writing for newspapers and magazines resulted in regular requests to be a guest health expert for all the daytime television shows that were filming in New York City, including *Rolonda, Sally Jessy Raphael, Gordon Elliot,*

Jenny Jones, Montel Williams and *Good Day New York*, as well as regular guest radio spots on *1010 WINS* news. This television exposure led me to the world of finance. I was hired to establish weight-loss centers to support the introduction of Redux, the first diet drug approved by the Food and Drug Administration (FDA) in more than 20 years. The FDA ultimately recalled Redux, but I continued to be fascinated by the world of drug development and the brilliant minds in this field that I met daily. I founded my corporate communications company, The Investor Relations Group (www.IRGnews.com), in December 1996.

For the past 16 years, I have worked closely with CEOs and top scientific and medical management teams from budding biotechnology, pharmaceutical and medical device companies (along with companies in other sectors as well). I've served on the board of the New York City chapter of the American Heart Association. Firsthand, I have witnessed cutting-edge science develop and have had plenty of opportunities to converse with leaders committed to healing the ills that are resulting from our modern diets and lifestyles.

On September 11, 2001, my husband, I and our then one-year-old daughter were living in downtown New York City, a few short blocks from the World Trade Center. Surviving the events of the day refocused me on countless levels. For one, I became more deeply intent on figuring out how to balance work and stress, to really appreciate life. I knew that being alive was a gift and I had better continue doing whatever was in my power to take excellent care of my "vehicle" (body!). I thought both my percentage of body fat and lung capacity could be improved. I had graduated from high school at 120 pounds, got married at 39 weighing 125, then watched my weight soar to 174 with both of my pregnancies and never again dip below 137 when I wasn't pregnant. I wanted to make sure I was in the best shape possible so I could live a long, vital life watching our two children grow up.

I continued testing all kinds of diet programs and exercise routines on myself, comparing before-and-after blood tests to assess the results, and always discussing notes with my brother Tom, who was analyzing his blood tests as well. For the majority of the time, I consumed a diet of grains, tubers, veggies, fruits and often a little low-fat dessert. People commented that I was "the healthiest, most energetic, most high-spirited person they knew."

As we moved into 2008 our experiments continued. We began testing the philosophy behind very low-calorie diets (VLCDs), what we now call "enlightened fasting," wondering if they really did eliminate hunger and moodiness. We experimented with walking as a sole form of exercise. We tried high-intensity weight lifting and then reduced it to mere one-minute routines. We continued to meditate and practiced transcendental meditation, Robert Monroe's Hemi-Sync combinations of sounds and voice, self-hypnosis, Reiki and everything else in the relaxation and stress-management fields.

Connecting the dots, with a little of this and a little of that, we began achieving startling reductions in our percentage of body fat that were rapid, astounding and very easy to achieve. Within only 20 days of implementing the techniques for food combining—or separation, actually, of proteins and fats from carbohydrates at any given meal—along with more activity vs. exercise, rest and relaxation, and a few other concepts we have shared, I became quite sleek and lean with more shapely muscles than ever as my weight quickly dropped from 137 pounds and 36% body fat to a startling 125 pounds and 22% body fat. With these results, coupled with the fact that

I was feeling quite fabulous, it was easy to keep going. As of this writing, I weigh-in fairly steadily at 117 pounds and have 13.5% body fat. I'm sleeker, leaner, and more toned than the day I graduated from high school and my blood work is impeccably perfect according to my personal physician, Dr. Fred Pescatore, author of *The Hamptons Diet* (and several other really great books). I am truly TurboCharged.

The TurboCharged steps can bring you comparable success. This is our goal and hopefully yours, too. The program is simply remarkable. It is built on a solid foundation of nutritionally sound scientific research. The testimonials throughout these pages from friends, relatives, colleagues and clients who were the earliest practitioners of this program document our claims. Their lives have been transformed, and you can enjoy the same results. We have streamlined the wealth of information from literally hundreds of books and thousands of articles down to the key facts and knowledge you need so you too can live in a sleek, lean, healthy, vibrant and physically strong body, while being better able mentally to handle any challenges that life throws at you, in ways you never could before. Follow our eight easy Steps and you too will experience the fabulosity of being TurboCharged!

This is a life-changing and exhilarating program. It will prove to you that you are capable of accomplishing whatever you desire. You will witness firsthand the many possibilities available to you and see that you can truly become whoever or whatever you want to be.

Supplemental Reading

All of the information within these pages has been culled from a lifetime of reading and personal experimentation. We "connected the dots" from the best-of-the-best. The end result is simply the most satisfying, rapid and comfortable program ever compiled for losing excess body fat permanently while simultaneously rebuilding health.

The following is a listing of some of our favorite books that helped us to formulate the program within these pages. They are in no particular order:

Orthopathy by Herbert M. Shelton (or any other book of his you can find!)

The Mucusless Diet Healing System by Arnold Ehret (or any other book you can find!)

The China Study by T. Colin Campbell, Ph.D.

Revitalize Your Life After 50 by Jack LaLanne (and any other book he's written!)

The Complete Triathlon Endurance Training Manual by Paul and Patricia Bragg (and all books by the Braggs)

The Wisdom of Milton H. Erickson (and any other books by M.H. Erickson)

TRANCE-formations by John Grinder and Richard Bandler

The Paleo Diet by Loren Cordain, Ph.D.

The Warrior Diet by Ori Hofmekler

The Primal Blueprint by Mark Sisson

The Hamptons Diet by Fred Pescatore, MD

The Atkins Diet by Robert Atkins, MD
Life Science System by T.C. Fry and others
Good Calories, Bad Calories by Gary Taubes
Eat for Health by William Manahan, MD
Dr. Carlton Fredericks' Low-Carbohydrate Diet by Carlton Fredericks
Neanderthin by Ray Audette with Troy Gilchrist
Sugar Blues by William Dufty
Lean Genes by Mark Davis
Slimdown for Life by Larry North
The Secret to Low Carb Success! by Laura Richard
Walk Yourself Thin by David Rives
The New Glucose Revolution by Brand, Miller, Wolever, Foster-Powell, Colagiuri
The Raw Food Body Building Training Manual by Charlie Abel
Fit for Life by Harvey and Marilyn Diamond
Eat To Live by Joel Fuhrman, MD
Raw Power! by Stephen Arlin
Conscious Eating by Gabriel Cousens, MD
Lean for Life by Clarence Bass (also *Ripped)*
The Okinawa Program by Willcox, Willcox & Suzuki
We Want to Live, the Primal Diet by Aajonus Vonderplanitz
The Carbohydrate Addict's Diet by Rachael and Richard Heller
Toxemia by John Tilden
Sweet Suicide by Gene Wright
The Soul Purpose by Ted Morter, Jr.
The HeartMath Solution by Doc Childre, Howard Martin with Donna Beech
Protein Power by Michael and Mary Dan Eades
The Family Nutrition Book by William and Martha Sears
The Doctor's Quick Weight Loss Plan by Irwin M. Stillman, MD

Support for Your TurboCharged Lifestyle

A ll over the country, individuals who have read TurboCharged and applied its principles are reaping the benefits. They are living examples of its effectiveness, and people in their communities are noticing. Although the comments vary, the most frequent questions are:

"How did you get so sleek and lean?"
"What kinds of workouts are you doing to stay so toned?"
"You look amazing!"
"What can I do to look as good as you?"
"What is your secret?"

You too will find that the response you will receive from others is wonderful and feels great. There may be the occasional negative comment, but remember, any comment or suggestion that does not support your best sleek, lean, healthy body is nothing other than sour grapes from someone who doesn't have the conviction that you do. They lack the determination and drive or the knowledge that has gotten you to awe-inspiring fabulosity. Don't listen to anything that is less than positive. Simply retort, "I'm not sure if that was a compliment, but I'll take it as one. I am proud of my accomplishments." Then refer them to the book!

Since you read this book, we know you are motivated to be lean and healthy for life. Your new knowledge and awareness, along with regularly implementing the TurboCharged steps, is all you will need to keep your new body and mind free from lapsing into your old fat ways of eating and living.

Countless individuals have been able to not only lose fat but also remain at their desired body composition goal by continuing to follow all of the steps of the TurboCharged program. Others find they like a little additional encouragement and community support. We have a few options for you to utilize to your heart's content.

www.TurboCharged.us.com

We want to help you keep your new lean and healthy body as a permanent and non-negotiable asset in your life. So in addition to referring to this book regularly, we invite you to join the TurboCharged community at www.TurboCharged. us.com. The website provides camaraderie in an online environment populated by others who, like you, have made the commitment to be sleek, lean and healthy. They no longer speak in terms of weight loss because they know that weight is merely a guideline. TurboCharged followers know that body fat is the issue. On the site you will get ongoing inspiration and ideas from us and be able to chat with others. You will be kept up-to-date on any new significant research that further validates and might ultimately be incorporated into the TurboCharged program.

On TurboCharged.us.com, you will also find all sorts of videos showing you new fun ways to incorporate activity into your life. You will also find delicious TurboCharged recipes, new mini-minute exercise ideas, chat, support and encouragement.

We hope you join us and invite your friends too. Please log in and visit often. We want to know you and cheer your success.

Dian and Tom log in regularly to provide insight and encouragement. The site provides a great forum to exchange ideas, discuss new trends, exchange recipes, ask questions about specific challenges or problems, and confirm which foods will contribute to your progress or not. For those of you who are into Cruise Control, there's plenty of daily talk and ideas on how to easily keep your fat loss permanent.

A Prototype Plan for Creating Your Own TurboCharged Community

Some people prefer human contact and commiseration for support. For you, we think that a support group just might be the answer. We want to provide you with some ideas that others have used to find like-minded TurboCharged advocates and a plan for making it effective.

A support group can provide its members with an opportunity for mutual growth and exchange. Members can share similar difficulties and feelings, and offer each other personal perspectives for resolving those difficulties or working through those feelings. Groups allow members the experience of learning that others face similar challenges. The exchange of knowledge and ideas promotes progress. Members can share their goals with the optimistic goals of others in the group so they can cheer each other's progress as they move forward as a community. A support group also provides encouragement when members encounter roadblocks, such as the occasional plateaus, and offers different strategies for success in meeting goals.

Support groups can be structured or informal. Group members can meet and decide on the preferred style. Often a group begins simply as a walking club with two members. Before long, others want to join the fun as they watch the fat dropping.

Some groups meet daily for walks and then weekly for conversation and comparing progress. Others establish a monthly meeting at a set location and often plan it at a restaurant that serves TurboCharged foods and they make it a communal dining experience.

Group leaders can establish a planned agenda, or the format can be kept casual. Regardless of the style, groups can provide tremendous support and therefore add to the likelihood of ongoing success for all those involved.

The most successful groups follow certain basic rules:

- The environment needs to be warm and non-judgmental so attendees are free to speak without embarrassment.

- The T.H.I.N.K. Rule should apply to any comments:

  T: Is the comment Thoughtful
  H: Is the comment Hurtful
  I: Is the comment Intelligent and in line with TurboCharged thinking
  N: Is the comment Necessary
  K: Is the comment Kind and encouraging of the success of others.

- Confidentiality must be respected. Personal disclosures must be kept confidential within the group.

- Medical opinions should be avoided. Medical advice is best dispensed by an individual's personal doctor after a good blood work-up.

- Personal experiences can be shared.

- Group leaders should rotate. By sharing the leadership task, everyone gets a sense of belonging and participation. Group leaders have a role of keeping the conversation moving, interesting and lively. No one individual should be allowed to dominate the discussion.

- Respect differences. It is important that group leaders encourage participation by all leaders—but don't force sharing. Some people learn by listening. Others will be more compelled to share regularly and often.

To get your group going, the steps are simple:

1) For starters, establish a leader if necessary; decide how that leadership will rotate.

2) Decide how large you want the group to be. As others see your success and you tell them to "read the book" your circle will likely grow. Look for members through like-minded friends, work, church, social groups and exercise facilities.

3) Choose how often you will meet: Daily for walks, weekly or monthly for chat.

4) Select a meeting place: A participant's home, church, restaurant, school, town hall or library.

5) Get everyone's contact information: name, telephone number, email address, mailing address.

6) Define your confidentiality and respect for other policies.

7) Determine the meeting format: Will food be allowed? Will each member be responsible for some aspect of a TurboCharged meal? Will the meeting be formal with an agenda or a casual gathering to chat? Will a specific topic be the focus of each meeting? Etc.

The most important aspects of any support group are the encouragement, support, community and progress reports of participants. Don't worry if your first meeting seems a little stilted. Lively discussion and exchange will increase as trust does within the community.

It is important to remember that you want to gain insight into your own behaviors, and receive and give feedback, support, knowledge and encouragement to each other. You aren't there to get "fixed" or "fix" others. We all come with our own perspectives (food-related and otherwise) and reach our own realities whenever we are ready.

One way of beginning is to have the group leader start with a discussion of "their story": a bit of past history struggling with weight and the end of that search once they began the TurboCharged program. No one should be forced to speak, but gently encouraged to share, if they are comfortable.

Conversations can get very lively if you ask participants to report the numbers from their body fat scales: Weight, Body Fat %, Water and Metabolic Age. As group members notice others not just getting leaner but younger, enthusiasm levels can really rise.

Members should be encouraged to share any material they determine to be relevant to the group: Maybe an article in a newspaper or magazine. Another failed fat celebrity who dieted yet gained it all back (yes—this is both fun gossip and motivating. You'll realize fame doesn't bring leanness!). Recipes that really fit the TurboCharged program. Products to enhance a TurboCharged lifestyle. Coupons regarding sales of TurboCharged supporting items. Community calendars and maybe information about a walk to raise money for a community event, etc.

"Buddies" are a common practice in certain support groups. Sometimes a buddy is selected for a period of time to help initiate a new member into the group. Buddies can be great. Sometimes buddies are a pain in the butt! Basically the concept of buddy is that you will each share your personal story more intimately. Having buddies is yet another decision for the group to decide to implement or not.

Support groups can provide great motivational enhancement to the TurboCharged program. We know people who have started them at their yoga center, office, church group and within countless other formats. Some members will be more competitive within the group than others and you can use them to everyone's inspirational advantage as you all watch them exceed their previously stated goals.

To be TurboCharged is a new way of life. It is the perfect holistic program that positions you for success not just today but for the rest of your life. With your support group in place, you and your group can all get and feel better, sleeker, leaner, healthier and more fabulous together!

Biographies

Dian Griesel, Ph.D., 50, is a serial entrepreneur and long-recognized health spokesperson. She founded The Investor Relations Group (www.IRGnews.com) in 1996. Today it is a nationally recognized, award-winning public relations and corporate communications firm. Dian lectures and writes on a variety of topics. She is a lifetime member of the International Association of Counselors and Therapists as well as the National Guild of Hypnotists. She has served on the Board of the New York Chapter of the American Heart Association.

In addition to TurboCharged, Dian is the author of: *Uncapped!, Capitalization Success, The 101 Platinum Plus Rules of Public Relations, Health Power, Health Power Recipes* and *Image Enhancement Weight Control and Hypnosis.* She has written health-related and other articles that have appeared in countless publications.

In the early 1990s, Dian was invited to appear as a regular health expert on *Sally Jessy Raphael, Gordon Elliot, Jenny Jones, Montel Williams, The Rolanda (Watts) Show, Good Day New York* and *1010 WINS news.* During this time, she also worked in private practice and taught continuing education classes in health, weight and stress management for the City University of New York and the NY Open Center.

In the 1980s, Dian was co-partner of Spotlite Marketing, a division of Spotlite Entertainment. She marketed corporate sponsorship deals for Jay Leno, Jerry Seinfeld, Yakov Smirnoff and many other top-tier acts.

Today Dian lives in Connecticut with her husband Rory and their two children.

Tom Griesel, 56, is the older brother of Dian and a true Renaissance man. When he wanted to learn to play guitar, he began by learning how to build his own instead of buying one. This enthusiasm for process has followed him throughout his life. Tom didn't just do triathlons—he trained, customized gear and hand-assembled the bike he rode on. He always wants to understand how and why things work the way they do. With this curiosity and passion, he has been studying health, wellness and longevity for over 30 years.

His lifetime interest in fitness, health and meditation has resulted in him becoming a Reiki Master as well as learning and regularly practicing Transcendental Meditation for over 20 years. He is one of the few fitness personalities who can actually demonstrate many impressive physical feats including, for example, doing 100+ push-ups in record time along with an equally impressive number of pull-ups as well.

Tom began his career in the marine industry, moved onto management of a public utility, founded an early vitamin-sale business, and co-founded a boutique investment banking firm that for the past 12 years financed pharmaceutical, biotechnology and other high-tech companies. In January 2010, he moved on again to finally live his dream of consulting and writing about wellness, fitness and fat loss.

Today Tom spends his time with Janet, his wife of 30+ years, along with their two Golden Retrievers, Jack and Clover, living in California, Arizona and Connecticut.

Made in the USA
Charleston, SC
22 March 2011